SUPERFOOD
Seagreens

I dedicate this book to so many of my colleagues and heroes who toil upon the seas and in labs, and those who pound the pavement, boiling up interest in this incredible food source. And I dedicate the recipes to a new generation of inspired cooks discovering new ingredients that improve our health and sustain the environments that sustain us. And a special thanks to Katy Rivera.

SUPERFOOD
Seagreens

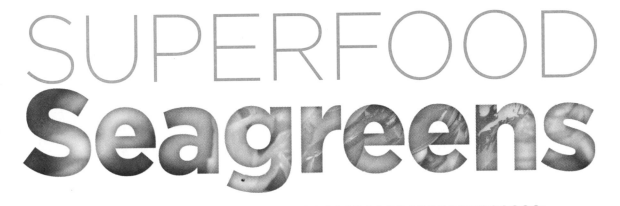

A Guide to Cooking with POWER-PACKED SEAWEED

BARTON SEAVER

STERLING
New York

STERLING
New York

An Imprint of Sterling Publishing
1166 Avenue of the Americas
New York, NY 10036

ISBN 978-1-4549-1739-7

Distributed in Canada by Sterling Publishing
c/o Canadian Manda Group, 664 Annette Street
Toronto, Ontario, Canada M6S 2C8
Distributed in the United Kingdom by GMC Distribution Services
Castle Place, 166 High Street, Lewes, East Sussex, England BN7 1XU
Distributed in Australia by Capricorn Link (Australia) Pty. Ltd.
P.O. Box 704, Windsor, NSW 2756, Australia

For information about custom editions, special sales, and premium and corporate purchases,
please contact Sterling Special Sales at 800-805-5489 or specialsales@sterlingpublishing.com.

Manufactured in Canada

2 4 6 8 10 9 7 5 3 1

www.sterlingpublishing.com

CONTENTS

Introduction vi

CHAPTER 1: Sustainable Seashores:
        The History and Future of Seagreens 1

CHAPTER 2: What Are Seagreens? 11

CHAPTER 3: The Power of Seagreens 19

CHAPTER 4: Equipping Your Kitchen and Pantry 33

CHAPTER 5: Buying and Preparing Seagreens 45

CHAPTER 6: Breakfast 55

CHAPTER 7: Snacks 69

CHAPTER 8: Sauces, Spices, and Sides 79

CHAPTER 9: Salads 99

CHAPTER 10: Soups 111

CHAPTER 11: Larger Dishes 125

CHAPTER 12: Breads, Muffins, and Desserts 135

CHAPTER 13: Frequently Asked Questions 141

Resources 150

About the Author 152

Acknowledgments 152

Photo Credits 153

Index 153

Throughout my life I've been fascinated by the marine world and all the tastes and textures it has to offer. As a young boy, I was captivated by the rocky shores and the tidepools and shallows in which I waded in discovery of an unknown world. This fascination with the ocean has always exerted a tidal pull on my creativity as a chef. And my focus has always been on seafood.

As seafood deliveries came to the back door of my restaurant, and as I pulled my line from the water, oftentimes there was a bit of seaweed tangled on the lure or nestled around food destined for the menu. For decades I overlooked seaweed as a nuisance or simply as packaging material no different from bubble wrap. But as I began to expand my culinary repertoire and became increasingly more interested in the tastes and textures of the ocean, it dawned on me that I had long overlooked an entire category of seafood. I began to experiment with the rockweed that came with deliveries of lobster and looked again at the strange ingredients found in packages in the Asian foods aisle at the grocery store. And I began to wonder how I could incorporate these ingredients into my cooking.

As my explorations continued, I found just what I expected—something completely new, wonderfully unique, charismatic, and almost endless in its creative applications. Although I found that seagreens were not an easy ingredient to introduce as a main course, they added vitality as a flavoring or garnish to my cooking, augmenting the subtle ocean flavors so prized in seafood. As I explored varieties of seagreens I'd previously overlooked, they soon claimed a permanent place in my cooking.

In keeping with my personality, I'm very curious about the provenance and nature of any and all products that I serve, and I began to investigate the sustainability, history, and nutritional aspects of seagreens. What I found, in almost every circumstance, was compelling information, prompting me to embrace these ingredients even more fully. From a cook's perspective, the characteristic umami flavors imparted by seagreens accentuate, highlight, and lend a richness of flavor to dishes. From a nutritional standpoint, they are as beneficial to our health as one could hope of any ingredient. And from a sustainability perspective, seagreens offer one of the greatest opportunities to create healthy, restorative, and delicious food systems.

While I understand there might be some hesitation from a cultural perspective to

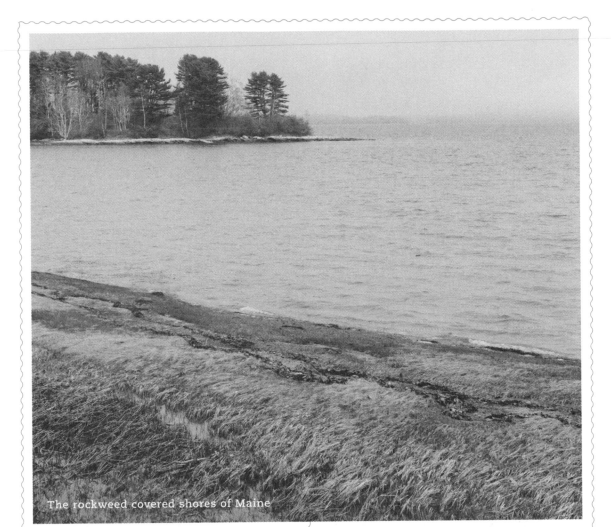

The rockweed covered shores of Maine

integrate seagreens into your diet, I encourage you to take a step back to reexamine a source of food that is not entirely unfamiliar: think of miso soup, sushi, and the commonly used agar (an extract of seagreens), and look at it in a new light to see the inherent value in these products, not only for the joy of discovery but also for the promise and practice of delicious and healthy eating. In so many ways, because they relate to the environment and our health and because they are so delicious and versatile, seagreens are without a doubt a superfood among superfoods.

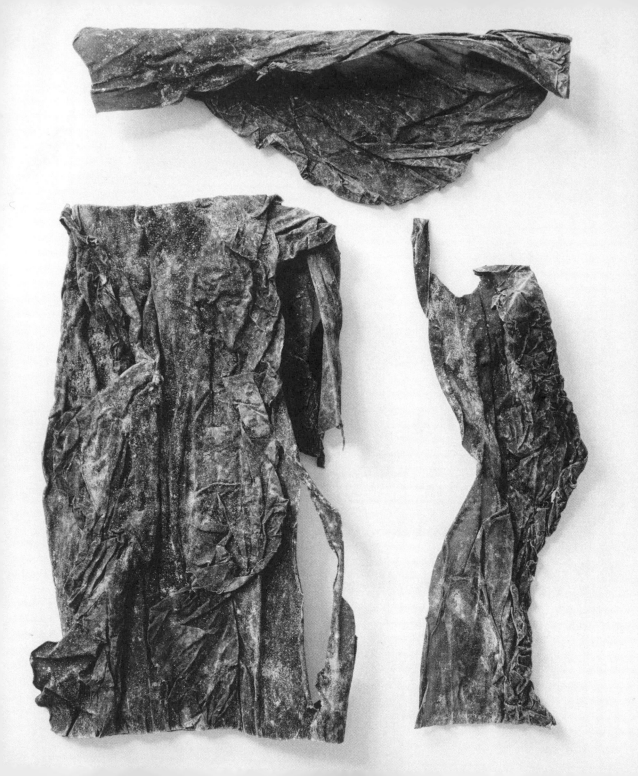

CHAPTER 1

SUSTAINABLE SEASHORES: THE HISTORY AND FUTURE OF SEAGREENS

For many of us, the smell of a sea-sweet breeze recalls charmed and treasured times relaxing along the coast. The salty tang of the crisp ocean scent is, in fact, punctuated by the smell of various seaweeds, what we call "seagreens" in this book. And while we've not traditionally associated that smell with food, its pleasant, clean, bracingly pure scent can be wonderfully evocative, enticing us to incorporate these greens into our diets. When seagreens are well treated in the kitchen, they can bring freshness and romance to any dish. In fact, some of my Japanese friends associate the comfort of home with the ever-present fragrance of a pot of seagreens simmering on the stove, a constant companion and a restorative tea to enjoy throughout the day. Just as the English are famous for enjoying a spot of tea, as much for the intake of caffeine as a celebration of tradition, a restorative broth of seagreens can bring an equal measure of comfort and enjoyment.

THE TABOO AGAINST SEAWEED

The common term for the oceans' bounty of plantlike algae is "seaweed," and because it grows near the seabed and is often obscured from our sight, we are often unaware of it. More often than not, our experience of seaweed is limited to the detritus washed upon the shore, the result of tide and storm. We perceive our pristine beaches as marred by chaotic clusters of unknown, tumbleweed-like plants that, once they begin to break down, punctuate the clean salt air with a whiff of low tide. Such seaweed is not used for food as seagreens must be freshly harvested. Additionally, for those of us who are fortunate to visit the ocean and wade into its embrace, patches of slippery seaweed can make for unsure footing. Fingerlike fronds of seaweed may coil discomfitingly around our legs, trailing our movements and making each step into the ocean an anxious advance into unknown territory, particularly for those of us who have any trepidation about the sea.

With so many inhibitions about seaweed, how can we reinvent our relationship with this long-neglected resource? I suggest we simply speak of seaweed in a different context. By calling them seagreens, we create a familiar association with them as food and embrace them as a culinary opportunity. It's high time to let go of our long-standing and ill-conceived dismissal of this incredible resource. Instead, let's further investigate seagreens and, in the process, discover a superfood that is at once sustainable and plentiful.

Throughout culinary history there are many examples of foods that were shunned because of a lack of familiarity with their true nature. The tomato, once nicknamed "poison apple" but now beloved as the edible icon of summer, is a perfect example. Lobster, once considered a fertilizer or food fit only for servants, is now revered as the pinnacle of luxury. Our preferences and tastes evolve. Through discovery and experience we gain familiarity and embrace foods we previously rejected. For example, how popular was kale ten years ago? Now it is de rigueur on restaurant menus and claims its own hashtags and cult followers. In my opinion, kelp is the new kale.

IT'S IN EVERYTHING

Seagreens in various forms and myriad varieties have long been a part of food production. Asian cultures have gathered and farmed seagreens for centuries, and their inclusion in many European cuisines has been a constant. The oceans are amazingly abundant and generous in the sustenance they afford us. Even though there is a long history of eating seagreens in the United States, they have never gained status as an iconic foodstuff, and while they may not appear on menus, they are everywhere in our food system. Seagreens contain natural thickening agents (some more than others), which, when extracted, can be used in an incredible number of food applications. Many of these products are part of our everyday diet. For example, carrageenan and agar are responsible for the smooth, luxurious texture of chocolate milk. They aid in creating the creaminess of candy bars, ice cream, toothpaste, and hand lotions—you name it. (See page 138 for a delicious traditional dessert recipe that highlights this velvetine texture.) Although seagreens and seagreen extracts are used in so many of the products we use every day, we don't consider them as part of our diet. But industrial uses of seagreens have paved the way for the development of seagreen

SEAGREENS, CLAMBAKES, AND OYSTER ROASTS

Wherever people have celebrated the sea's bounty, there are long and storied traditions of coastal cookouts, nearly all of which include seagreens. The most notable of these, in modern times, is the lobster bake or clambake of New England culinary fame. While the precise method of preparation varies from cook to cook, the basic idea is to steam a generous collection of diverse shellfish—clams, lobsters, and mussels, for example—over a slow, savory, and soulful fire. The first step is to build a driftwood fire in a deep hole in the sand. Next, a combination of delectable foods, including potatoes, corn, sausage—whatever you want—is added to the shellfish and nestled into a thick layer of seagreens that has been placed over the burning embers. More seagreens are strewn on top. The embers scorch the seagreens and create a smoky-sea sauna for the food. Although the process may take up to a couple of hours, the result is absolutely worth it, and the time waiting for dinner is well spent with friends and drinks. These events are truly unique celebrations, in beautiful places, of the tastiest of all ingredients.

The seagreen most commonly used for coastal cookouts is known as rockweed (or bladderwrack), a seagreen with long fronds and small air bladders along the stem, which pop and burst with seawater steam, imparting a wonderful summer scent to the food. If cooking dinner in a pit of sand for many hours just isn't in the cards for you, these flavors can be replicated at home: just add a good amount seagreens to a large pot of boiling water generously seasoned with salt, preferably sea salt. This will give beachside appeal to whatever you cook in the water. Don't think that you need the full array of clambake ingredients in order to enjoy the experience. The results are just as delicious if you cook corn or other vegetables such as asparagus, potatoes, or whole heads of broccoli along with the seafood. Any food that is typically steamed or boiled takes on a brilliant new personality and charisma when it is prepared with the salty, umami flavors of seagreens.

farming technologies that are promoting new opportunities for them to be grown for direct human consumption.

For many years, we've celebrated the incredible health benefits that come from a diversity of delicious plants and fruits. We've begun to understand and incorporate the idea that good health is built upon the pillar of a good diet. While many foods are nutritious—and delicious—a few are both truly compelling in the kitchen as well as storehouses of the vitamins and nutrients so essential to our health. Just as we have come to know these superfoods—quinoa from

South America, for example—it is no leap of faith that we should find another superfood readily available to us from the largest ecosystem on the planet.

Seagreens have long been an essential part of many coastal diets. Their medicinal and health benefits have been documented for centuries. One of the most exciting aspects of seagreens is that through them we have gotten to know an entirely new realm of textures, tastes, and flavors. Just imagine the vitality of the sea itself made into a salad. Seagreens are a superfood in ways beyond just their nutritional value. As our human population grows to nine billion (and even more, by some estimates) we desperately need to embrace new food production systems— and what an opportunity seagreens are! They are at once familiar, green, and leafy, adding texture and a unique flavor to any dish. One of the most compelling characteristics of seagreens is their rich umami flavor, the so-called "fifth flavor," best described as meaty and satisfying—a flavor that accentuates all others with which it is paired.

Given the familiarity of seagreens, finding comfortable and even innovative ways to incorporate them into our diet is an exercise in creativity. Who wouldn't love lasagna noodles soaked in family tradition and red sauce, made silken with ricotta cheese, punctuated with a slight bite of chile peppers, and layered with the charismatic flavor of seagreens, so full and rich on their own that they can easily augment or even replace the meat. The briny tang of seagreens lends charm to a guacamole, sour with fresh lime and aromatic with cilantro. Seagreens blend seamlessly to turn this familiar dish— a favorite for entertaining—into something innovative and nutritious (and certainly a centerpiece of conversation). There are so many delicious ways to incorporate seagreens into your diet. If you have any doubts, just think about the first time someone offered you kale. Well, my friend, I'm here to tell you that kelp is the new kale. So here's to your health!

SUSTAINABILITY AND PRODUCTION

Beyond being beneficial as part of the human diet, seagreens and their cultivation present an incredible opportunity to engage in food production systems that are environmentally sustainable (they do not damage and deplete the environments in which they are grown).

In fact, seagreen farming systems help to improve the health of the ecosystems in which they are produced. Seagreens are a product of the quality of the water in which they are grown. Much the same as land-based plants, seagreens also need nutrients.

In many cases, in our coastal environments there is an excess of nutrients, due to runoff from lawn fertilizers and other alterations to natural environments, which disrupt the land's ability to absorb these nutrients. As they flush into our waterways, they can create coastal ecosystems that are overnutrified. Now, don't mistake this as dangerous pollution, but rather simply an excess of natural nutrients. Too much of any nutrient in the water creates imbalances in the system.

Farming seagreens helps to remedy that. Seagreens thrive, given the ready availability of vital nutrients they need to grow. By absorbing this excess, they help restore biological balance and improve the quality of water, all the while producing delicious and affordable food. Just like land-based plants, they "breathe," absorbing carbon dioxide from the atmosphere. Farming seagreens actually converts 20 percent more carbon dioxide into plant matter than its production

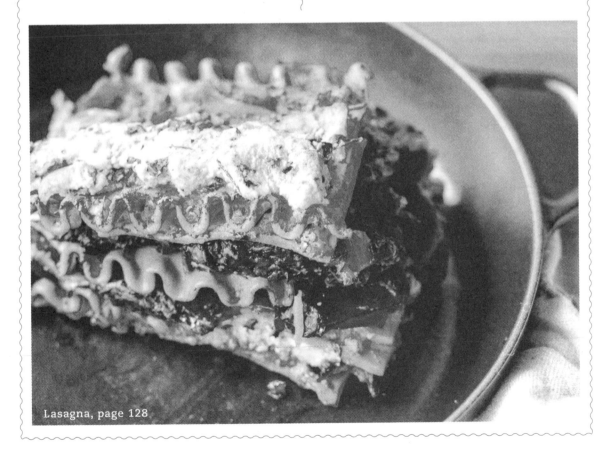

Lasagna, page 128

creates. This is known as a carbon sink. And while this is certainly not a cure-all for the increased carbon dioxide in our atmosphere, food production that has beneficial impacts is always welcome.

FARMING

Once seeded, seagreens require zero additional inputs. Their source of energy is natural, and the nutrients from which they grow are taken directly from the surrounding waters. They maintain the balance and resilience of coastal waterways and allow for incredible production levels. One of the other great advantages of seagreens is that unlike plants that grow on land, they do not have to expend any energy in order to counteract the effects of gravity. Buoyancy allows seagreens growth rates much greater than those of land-based plants, as the entirety of their energy is spent on growth rather than on competing against gravity.

FORESTS IN THE SEA

We are often familiar with seagreens as a product of the shoreline, clinging to rocks as the tide shifts. But seagreens also grow in immense forests in water fathoms deep. Growing dozens of feet long, the fronds gently swaying in the currents provide an essential habitat for countless sea creatures, much like tidal seagreens. In it, juvenile fish find safe places to hide from predators as they grow, and shellfish and other creatures find permanent homes there as well. In beautiful places such as Monterey Bay, California, immense kelp forests, visible at the surface, provide an incredible stage for us to view otters and seals, both at play and foraging for food. Because seagreens play such an essential role in the ecosystem, it's important to view and value them not just as an important addition to our diet but also as necessary parts of the ecosystems that ultimately support us.

GLOBAL INDUSTRY

Seagreens are a global industry, mainly centered in Asia, worth billions of dollars in international trade. Both wild harvest and, increasingly, farmed seagreens provide immense amounts of food and products for industrial uses, as a low-impact, even restorative method of food production. The economic and food production opportunities that seagreens offer will continue to grow, and that's a good thing. This increasingly important domestic industry is a major vehicle for job creation, and, even more importantly, it is fast becoming an accessible source of healthy and nutritious food.

THE LEAST DEADLY CATCH

When I was fourteen years old I dropped out of high school and headed out to sea. My first job on the boats was to stand on deck with a shotgun and shoot as many birds as possible before they stole the bait. You name it, I fished it: working the cod, salmon, tuna, and crab boats from Gloucester, Massachusetts, to Alaska's Bering Sea. I worked thirty-hour shifts on factory trawlers scraping the seafloor, ripping up entire ecosystems; I fished illegally at night in protected waters and threw thousands of pounds of dead bycatch back into the sea; I pillaged the oceans, working for one of the most unhealthy, destructive forms of food production on the planet.

Eventually, the destruction became too much to bear. I wanted to spend my life working at sea, but the industry was charting a shortsighted voyage to ruin. After the cod stocks crashed back in my home of Newfoundland, a whole generation of us decided to chart a new course toward sustainability. We dreamed of being ocean stewards, not pillagers. So I began searching. First, I headed off to salmon farms in Canada to try my hand at aquaculture, which promised to be the answer to overfishing and feeding the planet. But when I arrived I found yet another unsustainable industry. On the salmon farms we pumped our fish full of antibiotics and polluted local waterways with pesticides. We were growing what I considered neither fish nor food.

Once again disillusioned, I kept searching. My journey took me to Long Island Sound, where there was a program to lease shellfishing grounds to young commercial fishermen under the age of forty. I leased twenty acres, started oysters, and then slowly, with many experiments and failures, transitioned the farm into one of the first three-dimensional ocean farms in the country. At its core, my model changed our relationship to the seas: turning fishermen into ocean farmers and restoring rather than depleting our oceans.

My farming design is simple: picture it as a three-dimensional underwater garden, where seaweed, mussels, and scallops grow on floating ropes at the top of the water column, stacked above oysters and clams below. I grow multiple species to foster a sea-basket approach to ocean farming, rather than promoting a monoculture. On a mere twenty acres I grow six different species—kelp, gracilaria, oysters, mussels, scallops, and clams, as well as sea salt.

While shellfish have had their turn as both a delicacy and a staple food source in our country for hundreds of years, the seaweed that we grow alongside these foods is less familiar. It shouldn't be, though. A native seaweed like nori contains more vitamin C than orange juice, more calcium than milk, and more protein than soybeans. And it might surprise those of you who are on the hunt for omega-3s to learn that many fish do not create these heart-healthy nutrients—they consume them. By eating the plants that fish eat, we get the same benefits. Some restaurants, such as Beyond Sushi in Manhattan, have already crafted entire menus around these sea vegetables, and a bevy of gourmet chefs are working on recipes to make locavores swoon.

In a sense, we're working to forge a new form of ocean cuisine built around ocean vegetarianism, which moves plants to the center of the plate and pushes wild fish to the edges. Scaled up, the potential impact on our food system is mind-blowing. In a three-hundred-foot by three-hundred-foot plot, we can grow twenty-four tons of seaweed in five months. Creating a network of small seaweed farms equaling the size of Washington State could provide enough food to feed the world. Of course we're not all going to become ocean vegetarians, but it shows our model can have a real impact on our stressed food systems.

The best news is that our farms do more than grow food. In every sense they restore rather than deplete. Matched up against land-based farming, these new ocean farms win every time. Seaweed and shellfish require no additional inputs—no land, no fertilizer, no fresh water—and since they grow three-dimensionally, they use space more efficiently than their land-based counterparts.

Shellfish and seaweed also act as filters, drawing nitrogen out of seawater—the primary objective of the Clean Water Act. While nitrogen is an important nutrient for humans, excess nitrogen from residential and agricultural runoff into the Long Island Sound regularly triggers large-scale algal blooms that deplete oxygen levels, kill marine life, and force beach closures. With a single oyster filtering up to fifty gallons of water a day, even small farms can have a measurable impact on water quality. Our mussels have one thirtieth the carbon footprint of industrially produced chicken; our farms function as artificial reefs and storm-surge protectors during hurricane season; and our kelp soaks up five times more carbon than land-based plants.

Finally, ocean farms open both new and old pathways for economic development. A decentralized system of small-scale operations could revitalize life along the shoreline, first by creating new green jobs on farms and alternative energy industry, and then, as the sea recovers, perhaps opening up old fisheries and bringing back traditional means of making a living.

To scale this restorative ocean economy, we created GreenWave, a nonprofit designed to replicate our model around the country. We run an apprentice program to train unemployed fishermen to be ocean farmers. Our school-to-farm program helps students learn new skills, so they can participate in the emerging blue-green economy. We build infrastructure, ranging from hatcheries to seafood innovation hubs, so that ocean farmers can share rescues and develop new value-added food products and thereby capture more of the value chain. We even have a seagreens food truck in the works to move our farmers' produce beyond restaurants and into the streets.

Humans depend on our oceans for survival. Every other breath we breathe comes from sea life. Three and a half billion people depend on seafood as a primary source of protein. We can't survive as a species without our oceans. We need to save our seas to save ourselves.

Despite the perils of overfishing, climate change, and acidification, I am hopeful and believe that we are on the brink of a blue revolution. I look out into the future and see a network of small-scale ocean farms like mine dotting our coastlines, surrounded by conservation zones, growing healthy local food while reducing carbon emissions and restoring our ocean ecosystems. After years of despair, I'm now convinced there is hope for saving our seas and our planet. Together we can turn the tide. So cook up a plate of seagreens and start a new blue revolution!

—BREN SMITH
GreenWave Executive Director and
Owner of Thimble Island Oyster, Co.

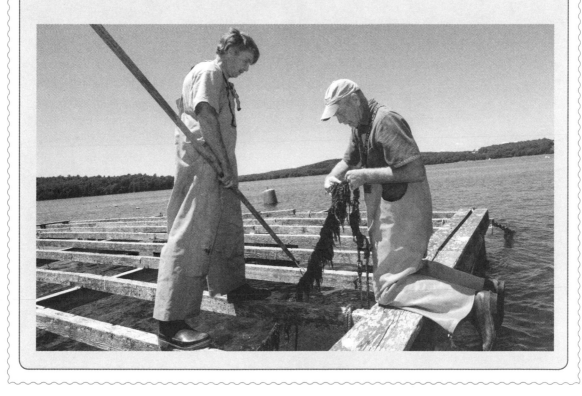

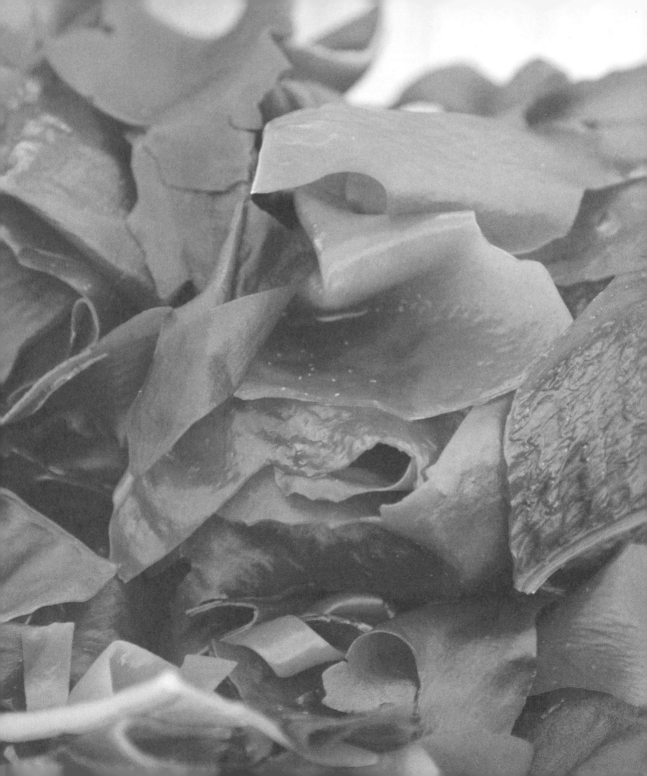

CHAPTER 2

WHAT ARE SEAGREENS?

Seagreens are algae, a term that designates a large group of organisms that are related to plants. The number of species in this group is estimated to be in the range of multiple millions. Algae grow in both freshwater and saltwater and are found in two forms: microalgae and macroalgae. All of the species in this book are macroalgae and come from the sea.

Of the thousands of known varieties of seaweeds or marine algae, we count only a few hundred in the category of seagreens. There are many varieties of kelp, for instance, a number of which fall under the category of culinary use and can be purchased whole, fresh, frozen, and dried, or as flakes and powders.

Seagreens do not need to grow roots because their cells, which are exposed to the surrounding water, absorb all the nutrients they need. Like plants, algae are photosynthetic and require sunlight in order to live; thus their range is typically found near the shore, where light penetrates the water. In many cases, seagreens may even be exposed for part of the day, when the tides roll out, giving them direct exposure to life-sustaining light.

This book explores only a few of these species, even though most seagreens are edible. However, not all of them are available in the marketplace—at least not yet. In this book, the options have been pared down to reflect what is currently and commonly available in some health food and grocery stores. Almost any seagreen can easily be ordered online, if you can't find what you're looking for at the store. Please see page 150 for a list of currently available products and where to find them.

A LITTLE GOES A LONG WAY

Currently there are no dietary recommendations regarding the consumption of seagreens. As with all things, moderation is a good idea, especially given the known content of iodine in seagreens. Aim for a little every day, rather than a lot once in a while.

COMMON SEAGREENS

Hundreds of species of seagreens are consumed worldwide. The categories below represent the most common forms of seagreens that can be found in markets (and online) and describe their general culinary characteristics and uses.

BROWN ALGAE

There are thousands of species of brown algaes, and almost all are marine based. They are generally the largest of the algaes and can survive in colder waters. They are named for their brown color, imparted by the xanthophyll pigment fucoxanthin. The presence of this pigment blocks the more brightly colored chlorophylls and beta-carotene.

THE KELPS, KOMBU

Kelps make up the majority of brown algae species.

Winged Kelp, *Alaria esculenta*

This beautiful, thick-ribbed, frond-like seagreen is found in intertidal and nearshore areas. Also known as alaria and Atlantic wakame, winged kelp is mostly sold in dried form and lends a subtle background flavor and a mild saltiness to Basic Dashi Broth (see page 111) and other stocks. Commonly known as kombu and lady kelp (my favorite name for this versatile seagreen), winged kelp has a high umami content (see "Umami and MSG" on page 14), thus strengthening and making bold the presence of companion flavors. No wonder *Alaria esculenta* means "edible wings!" As a dried seagreen, it is great for rehydrating (see page 49) and enjoying as a side dish or salad, especially when it is rehydrated with vinegar (see pages 49–50). The acidity really boosts the floral and delicate flavor of the seagreens. It is ideal dried and crumbled over salads or added to sautéed vegetable dishes just before serving. More than any other seagreen, it retains its texture, making it a good choice for adding a bit of crunch to warm dishes, such as Zucchini and Seagreens "Spaghetti" with Garlic (see page 129).

> ### DID YOU KNOW?
>
> Kelp can supply the full daily requirements of carotenoids, vitamin A, vitamin B_1, vitamin B_2, vitamin B_6, vitamin B_{12}, vitamin D, and pantothenic acid.

SPIRULINA

Spirulina, often called blue-green algae, is related to seagreens and has similar nutritional components. As a dietary supplement (including tablets and powder), spirulina has long been a favorite of the health food movement, as it is easy to integrate into foods and supplies great nutrition (for example, spirulina is a complete protein that contains all essential amino acids) without altering flavor too much. In this book, seagreens are treated as whole ingredients, not as additives, and celebrated for their versatility and flavor.

Wakame, *Undaria pinnatifida*

This is the seagreen that has become familiar as the bright green salad accompaniment to sushi. The near neon-green color of wakame, in this preparation, is achieved by lightly salting the blanched blades (what we would call the leaves) of the seaweed. Some commercial seagreen salads are heavily laden with food coloring, so it is worth checking the label. Wakame salad is commonly flavored with a bit of chile for a complementary bite and sesame oil for a deeply round and rich flavor. I like to toast wakame and crumble it over salads and main dishes to give them a crispy texture and rich flavor.

Sugar Kelp, *Saccharina latissima*

Sugar kelp, also called kombu, is probably the most common of the seagreens that you are likely to use. That's a good thing, as it is, to my taste, the most versatile product. Sugar kelp is so named due to the natural sugars that give this seagreen a floral and fruity hint. It is delicious as either a fresh or frozen product and is used as a stand-in for spinach or kale in smoothies. It is both harvested from the wild and farmed in North America, and it is the seagreen variety that will most likely break through as the leading product of this emerging industry. Sugar kelp is the principal variety I use for broths. When dried, the fronds of this seagreen can be very thick, while the rehydrated product gains good texture and a snap, almost like that of a green bean. This kelp lends itself well to use in salads and can be successfully rehydrated in a broth, then chopped into small pieces and incorporated as an ingredient beyond just the flavored liquid. I think it pairs particularly well with onions as a complementary sweetness; the spicy kick of a raw onion can really flatter the broad flavor of this seagreen and bring it more into focus.

UMAMI AND MSG

Umami, a flavor that occurs naturally in many foods, was identified in Japan in around 1910 by Kikunae Ikeda. In Japanese umami roughly translates as "delicious taste" or "pleasant savory taste." In some cultures, umami is referred to as the fifth taste, distinct from sweet, sour, bitter, and salty, revealing just how important this flavor is to cuisine as well as to our sensory understanding of taste. Umami is found in a range of common foods, including seagreens, the ingredient in which it is probably the most prevalent, though nuts, avocados, and especially mushrooms all contribute this foundational flavor to the dishes in which they are included.

Although the term "umami" is a relatively recent addition to the Western culinary lexicon, our appreciation of its qualities goes as far back as the first foods cooked over fire. Defined by a meaty and woodsy flavor, umami provides deep-layered complexity to ingredients that can be accentuated through various cooking techniques, such as searing.

As a chemical additive, umami has been widely applied through the use of the food additive MSG (monosodium glutamate, also known as sodium glutamate), made popular in decades past. While MSG has since proven to be a less-than-desirable additive, the MSG in umami-rich foods, such as seagreens, occurs naturally and is devoid of the potentially adverse effects of chemically created MSG seasoning.

Bullwhip Kelp, *Nereocystis luetkeana*

Found on the Pacific Coast of North America, this giant variety of kelp is delicious when dried and then toasted. The long stipe (what most of us would erroneously call the stem) makes a perfect pickle, though it needs to be sliced thin, as the vertical fibers can be very tough to chew. These pickles have an incredible snappy texture, and the ring-shaped stipes with a completely hollow center are fun to work with. *Nereocystis* means "mermaid's bladder" in Greek.

Rockweed, *Fucus vesiculosus*

Rockweed, though not a kelp, is a member of the brown algae family. Also known as bladderwrack, this is the seaweed you are probably most familiar with, as its frilly, flowerlike fronds punctuated by little bubbles (air bladders that keep them afloat) are commonly found along the shores of beaches and tourist areas. Rockweed is harvested in the wild and is not usually suitable for direct consumption. Only the very tender tips of fresh rockweed are well suited for this—

sautéed in a little bit of butter, for example, or fried in light cornmeal or tempura batter. The remaining fronds are often used fresh as part of the steaming process in a clambake or lobster boil. They impart a heavy perfume and umami boost to seafoods and provide a good amount of salt for the cooking water. Sausages, potatoes, and corn that are boiled with rockweed take on a character that elevates flavors and even textures to a higher level of succulence.

Dried forms of rockweed, whether it's the tender tips or the more leathery lower fronds, are sometimes used for smoking, lending a rich, cherry-mahogany flavor to meats and a beautiful walnut hue to seafoods. Unlike the sweet fragrance of almost any wood used for smoking, rockweed imparts aromas of salty brine, coastal air, and the inimitable scent of a driftwood fire on the beach—a perfect sunset scene. How better can I sell this to you? Smoking seafood with rockweed (along with your favorite accompaniments, whether it's potatoes or corn or whatever) is really worth trying. The rockweed also makes a fun popping sound when you throw it onto the embers of a charcoal fire—and it smolders for a surprisingly long time.

RED ALGAE

The pigments phycoerythrin and phycocyanin give red algae their color and name. There are more than 6,500 known species of red algae, most of them marine. Several red algae are suitable for consumption, the most popular being nori, dulse, and Irish moss.

IRISH MOSS, CHONDRUS CRISPUS

This species of red algae, also called carrageen moss, grows year-round in intertidal and nearshore areas of the northern Atlantic.

ROCKWEED: DID YOU KNOW . . . ?

- Much like grasses that grow in intertidal zones, rockweed provides a habitat for many species, including crustaceans, mussels, snails, and juvenile fish.

- The presence of rockweed is a good indicator of water quality because it tends to grow in abundance in nutrient-balanced water.

- Individual rockweeds generally live eight to ten years but can get much older!

Carrageenan, a common food additive used as a thickener and emulsifier to improve the consistency of some processed foods, such as yogurt and ice cream, is extracted from this and other red algae. Its flavor is so mild, it is hardly apparent at all.

DULSE, *PALMARIA PALMATA*

When fresh, this dark purple seagreen is beautiful, with a dense texture and brilliant sheen. Dulse can be used directly in myriad dishes. When it is dry, dulse takes on a particular potency that requires a little loving. Its somewhat dark and brooding flavor is great as an addition to full-flavored soups, such as a minestrone, where the brilliant flakes partner well with a mix of robust vegetables. Dulse crisps nicely into chips. It is widely available from Maine Coast Sea Vegetables™ in dried leaves that have been smoked over applewood, complementing their leathery texture and imparting a whiff of rich bacon. Dulse is also a good source of protein, thus making it even better as a substitute for meat. Broths made from dulse are well flavored and best used with other full-flavored ingredients. If you were to braise a shortrib, for example, you'd be better off using a dulse broth rather than a light kombu dashi. The bold, rustic flavors of dulse are a particularly good counterpoint to the acid tang of goat cheese.

LAVER, *PORPHYRA UMBILICALIS*, NORI

Found in intertidal and nearshore areas, this seagreen is principally and best known as nori. Compounds found in *Porphyra* offer protection from UV rays. Varieties harvested in North America, known as Atlantic nori, are not the same species as the Japanese variety, *Pyropia yezoensis*, although they are related and can be used interchangeably. Laver is the among the most nutritious of the seagreens, containing vitamins B_1, B_6, B_{12}, C, and E, as well as protein, fiber, iron and other minerals, and trace elements. Of the seaweeds, it also has the lowest iodine content.

In its dried form, nori is a perfect product to crumble over and mix into salads, and to blend with goat cheese or cream cheese as a spread for appetizers. Dried nori retains its texture for a short time before it softens considerably, so it is best to add it to dishes immediately before serving. Nori has recently become very popular, sold in thin chips and flavored with various seasonings, such as garlic, sesame, and wasabi, to name just a few. Many people I know think of nori as a bit of a "gateway" seagreen because its flavors and textures are so accessible. The larger, green-turning-to-black sheets of nori that are used as wrappers in maki sushi (or sushi roll) preparations are familiar to almost everyone now. In its unprocessed form, nori is quite leathery and elastic in its bite, although after the initial snap, it has a wonderfully chewy texture, not unlike that of a fruit leather. Nori has a mild nutty flavor, which is enhanced with toasting. Try dry-toasting nori in a pan over low heat until it turns slightly green and fragrant.

AN EVOLVING STORY

The science behind the nutritional benefits of seagreens is still being explored. Please check the resources on page 150 to find links for the most up-to-date information.

GREEN ALGAE

Green algae is so named because of the green color imparted by chlorophyll, a green color highlighted by quantities of beta-carotene (a yellow pigment). Many scientists believe plant life originated from green algae. These algae are mostly aquatic but can also be found in terrestrial environments, growing in the soil, on trees and rocks, and even in symbiotic relationships with fungi or animals.

SEA LETTUCE, ULVA LACTUCA

This brilliant green, delicately textured, yet chewy seagreen has a deep, rich flavor, similar to spinach, with a briny kick. When sea lettuce is toasted (dried in an oven) or sautéed in butter or bacon fat (even better), the flavor softens and it becomes a delightful snack or side dish. When flaked, sea lettuce looks like dried oregano and adds a beautiful green fleck (not to mention powerful nutrition) to all kinds of beverages, whether it's a smoothie or a Bloody Mary. It's also the best of the seagreens to use as an addition to seasonings such as Herbes de Provence or Creole Grill Seasoning (page 87).

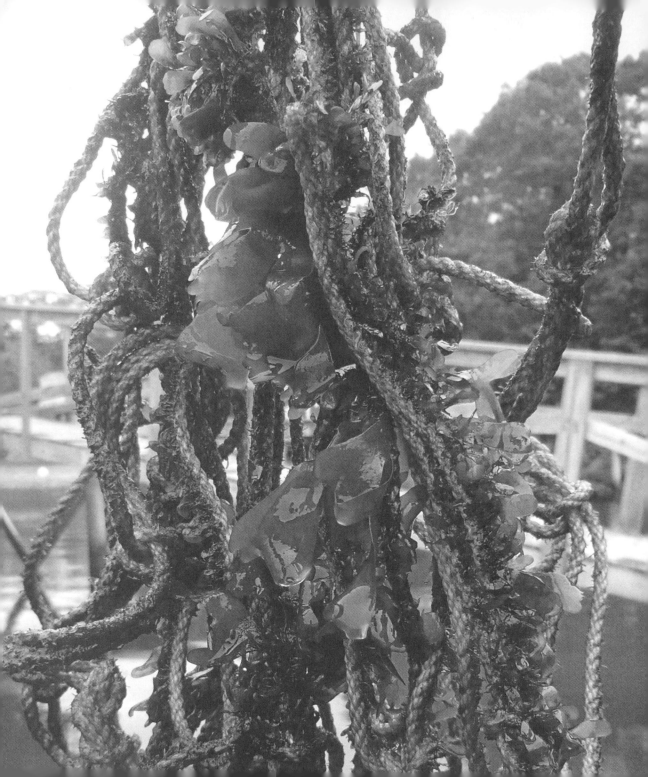

CHAPTER 3

THE POWER OF SEAGREENS

Seagreens are a true superfood. They are amazingly rich in many essential components of a healthy diet and contain more than twenty-five vitamins and more than fifty minerals, including vitamin A, vitamin C, vitamin B_6, vitamin B_{12}, folate, vitamin D, calcium, potassium, magnesium, phosphorus, iron, protein, iodine, sulfur, sodium alginate, sterols, and more. The amounts of each mineral range in quantity, but overall, they contain many times more minerals than land-grown plants. Ounce for ounce, they have more vitamins and minerals than many typical food sources. Seagreens are versatile and delicious, gluten-free, fat-free, and paleo, vegetarian, and vegan friendly. And seagreens, in their various forms, can be incorporated into nearly every style and method of cooking to increase flavor and nutrition in everything ranging from breakfast foods and snacks to soups and stews. Because seagreens are such nutritional powerhouses, you need to eat only a little to get a lot of benefits. In order to get the most nutritional return from eating seagreens, try to consume a little bit (half cup of fresh or frozen or half ounce of dried seagreens) at least three times a week. Once you get into the habit of adding seagreens to your repertoire, it'll be easy and delicious and you'll wonder what you've been doing without them for all these years.

VITAMIN A

A one-cup serving of raw nori seaweed provides over 75 percent of the recommended daily allowance (RDA) of vitamin A. It is essential to eye health, prevention of night blindness, promotion of skin health, and processing iron to produce red blood cells' immune function. Vitamin A comes in two forms: retinoids from animal products and beta-carotene from plant- or algae-based sources, such as seagreens. Vitamin A is a fat-soluble vitamin (consume it with fats for optimal absorption). Try adding a bit of olive oil to seagreens for maximum vitamin A absorption, as well as rich flavor.

NON-SEAGREEN SOURCES: Sweet potatoes, carrots, dark leafy greens, winter squashes, lettuce, dried apricots, cantaloupe, bell peppers, fish, liver, and tropical fruits.

VITAMIN C

Vitamin C is found in all varieties of seagreens and is essential for cell growth, a healthy immune system, and healing wounds. Vitamin C is also necessary for protein synthesis to create skin, tendons, ligaments, and blood vessels. A one-cup serving of raw nori seaweed provides more than 50 percent of the RDA of vitamin C.

Sometimes more is better: combining seagreens with other fruits and vegetables that contain high amounts of vitamin C aids in the absorption of iron, which can be found in plants such as seaweed, beans, and spinach.

NON-SEAGREEN SOURCES: Almost all fruits and vegetables contain some vitamin C. The highest concentrations can be found in cantaloupe, citrus, tropical fruits like mango, pineapple, kiwi, berries of all kinds, broccoli, brussels sprouts, cauliflower, green and red peppers, leafy greens, sweet and white potatoes, tomatoes, and squash.

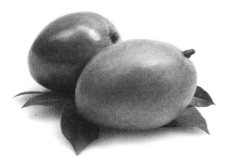

DID YOU KNOW?

In 1747, a discovery was made aboard a Royal British Navy ship that had been at sea for almost two months. Several sailors began to show symptoms of an unknown malady: their gums were sore, their teeth were falling out, and their legs were bruising. The sailors were so beset by pain and misery that they were unable to eat.

A doctor aboard the ship, Dr. James Lind, took a particular interest in this and began a clinical nutrition study of twelve of the afflicted sailors. Six groups of two sailors each were started on a regimen of different foodstuffs, including vinegar, barley water, and orange and lemon juice, among others. After just six days, five of the groups, which had not been given citrus, showed zero signs of recovery and their symptoms had worsened. On the other hand, the sixth group, which consisted of men who had been given citrus, had almost completely recovered. From that time on, every British sailing vessel carried citrus fruit onboard to stave off scurvy, a sickness that was later found to be caused by deficiency of vitamin C. As it turns out, seagreens are a great source of vitamin C. If only those sailors had known, they could easily have harvested seagreens to cure what was ailing them.

B VITAMINS

B vitamins, which allow us to create energy from the food we eat and are essential in creating red blood cells, can be found in all seagreens. Research indicates that some B vitamins may reduce heart disease. Other non-seagreen sources of B vitamins include proteins such as fish, poultry, meat, eggs, and dairy products; leafy green vegetables; beans; and peas. Try combining these complementary foods with seagreens to get the most vitamin B bang for the buck.

Vitamin B_6, vitamin B_{12}, and folate are found in relatively high quantity in seagreens. Vitamin B_{12} is not generally found in plant form, making seagreens particularly important to a healthy vegan diet, as vitamin B_{12} is essential to our nervous system and blood cell health. It is also necessary to create DNA, the genetic building blocks of all cells. NON-SEAGREEN SOURCES OF B_{12}: Meat (particularly beef liver), poultry, fish (clams in particular), eggs, milk, and other dairy products.

FOLATE

Folate, one of the B vitamins, is found in almost all seagreens. A one-cup serving of raw nori seaweed provides more than 25 percent of the RDA of folate. Folate is essential for creating DNA and other genetic material, as well as cell division, and is particularly important for women of childbearing age. Folate deficiency during pregnancy can increase the risk of having a baby with neural tube defects, such as spina bifida, as well as increasing the risk of a premature or low-birth-weight baby. Regular consumption of seagreens can prevent such a deficiency. NON-SEAGREEN SOURCES: Folate is found in vegetables such as asparagus, brussels sprouts, dark green leafy vegetables, oranges and orange juice, nuts, beans, peas, and fortified grain products. Small amounts of folate are found in meats (with the exception of beef livers, which are quite high

> ### B VITAMINS: DID YOU KNOW. . . ?
>
> - Vitamin B_6 may reduce nausea and vomiting during pregnancy.
>
> - Vitamin B_{12} deficiency can cause fatigue, weakness, constipation, unexplained weight loss, loss of appetite, and, in extreme forms, megaloblastic anemia. Eating seagreens can help prevent B_{12} deficiency and its resulting symptoms.
>
> - In older adults, vitamin B_{12} may lower levels of homocysteine, a contributor to dementia.

in folates), poultry, seafood, eggs, and dairy products. Combine any of these foods with seagreens to increase the available amount of folate for maximum absorption.

VITAMIN D

Vitamin D is essential for healthy bones. The body needs vitamin D in order to absorb calcium (this is why milk is frequently fortified with vitamin D). Vitamin D is found naturally in only a few foods, such as seagreens, and most of the vitamin D Americans get is through fortified foods. Some studies link vitamin D deficiency with an increased risk of diabetes, hypertension, and multiple sclerosis. Deficiencies in vitamin D can cause bone ailments such as osteomalacia, osteoporosis, and, in children, rickets. Studies indicate that vitamin D may reduce the risk of some cancers, including colon, prostate, and breast cancer.

Consumption of vitamin D through food sources, including seagreens, may help prevent these ailments.
NON-SEAGREENS SOURCES: Beef liver, cheese, seagreens, egg yolks, mushrooms, and fatty fish, such as salmon, tuna, and mackerel.

CALCIUM

Calcium is essential for bone health and muscular function. Most Americans do not get enough calcium from their diets. Studies indicate that proper calcium intake can reduce the risk of developing high blood pressure (hypertension). Calcium cannot be produced by the body and must be consumed in the foods we eat. Seagreens are a great source of dietary calcium. A one-cup serving of fresh kelp contains almost half of your RDA of calcium—more than one eight-ounce serving of 1 percent lowfat milk!
NON-SEAGREENS SOURCES: Calcium can also be found in dairy products, dark leafy greens, and the soft bones of fish, such as canned anchovies and sardines.

VITAMIN E

Seagreens contain vitamin E in the highly absorbable form of alpha-tocopherol. Vitamin E is a fat-soluble vitamin that acts as an antioxidant. It is critical to the production of red blood cells and allows the body to use vitamin K. Vitamin E deficiency can cause liver and kidney problems in the long term. Studies have shown that vitamin E contributes to a lower risk of heart disease and may reduce the risk of stroke in postmenopausal women. Some studies link vitamin E to cancer prevention and reduced development of Alzheimer's disease. Many more studies show that vitamin consumption from foods, such as seagreens, is much more effective than taking supplements.

NON-SEAGREEN SOURCES: Wheat germ, liver, eggs, nuts, seeds, cold-pressed vegetable oils, dark green leafy vegetables, sweet potatoes, avocado, asparagus, and yams are all good sources of vitamin E.

VITAMIN K

Vitamin K is a fat-soluble vitamin responsible for blood clotting. Vitamin K can be created by the bacteria found in the gastrointestinal tract lining, but consumption via food sources is necessary as part of a healthy diet. Kelp is particularly high in vitamin K. A one-cup serving of fresh kelp contains more than 60 percent of the RDA.

NON-SEAGREEN SOURCES: Green leafy vegetables, brussels sprouts, broccoli, cauliflower, cabbage, fish, liver, meat, and eggs.

IODINE

Seagreens have high quantities of iodine, a nutrient that is essential to our health. Iodine helps regulate our thyroid function. Women with underactive thyroids may show increased function with frequent consumption of seagreens. Iodine acts as a thyroxin precursor, regulating metabolism. It also helps prevent infection, protects us from environmental radiation, and combats the buildup of free radicals.

Currently in the United States more people are iodine deficient than iodine sensive. Thankfully, kelp is one of the most concentrated, naturally occurring sources of iodine. (Eat up!) Other sources of dietary iodine include seafood, dairy products, and plants grown in iodine-rich soil. However, if you have any concerns regarding increased intake of iodine, please consult your doctor.

IODINE: DID YOU KNOW. . . ?

* Beginning in 1924, acting on a recommendation by the US government, iodine was added to table salt sold by the Morton Salt Company™. Today, iodized salt is the main source of dietary iodine.

* Some studies show that patients undergoing radiation or chemotherapy seem to benefit from regular consumption of seaweed broth, perhaps due to the nutrient content, specifically iodine. Patients consuming seaweed broth report less frequent and less intense adverse reactions to treatment, easier recovery, and a general sense of wellness.

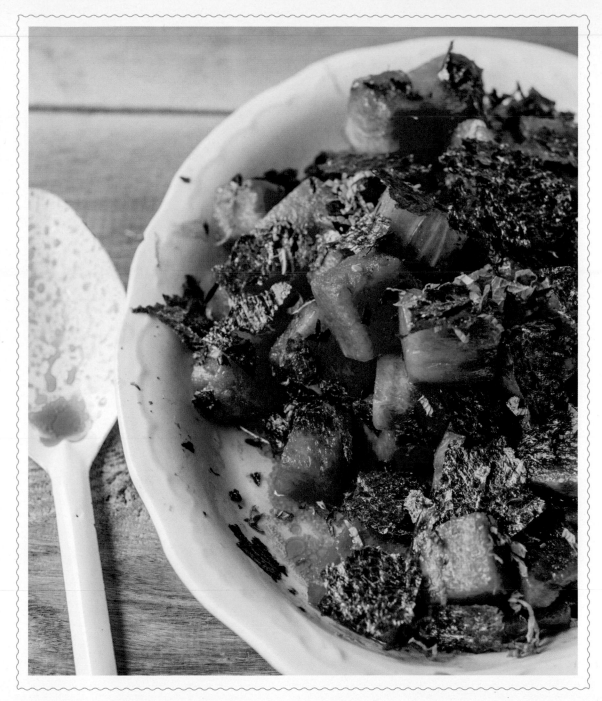

Watermelon Salad with Lime, Mint, and Nori, page 100

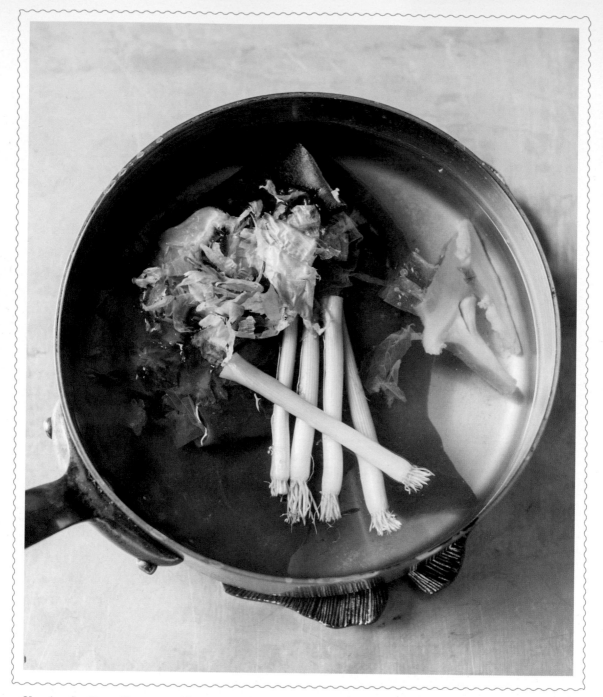

Kombu, Scallion, Ginger, and Bonito for Aromatic Dashi Broth, page 112

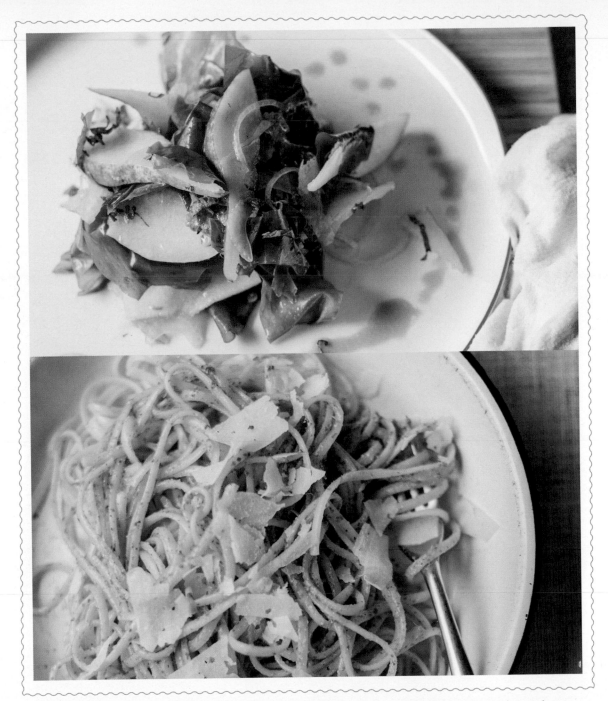

TOP: Pear and Herbs over Seagreens Salad, page 106 BOTTOM: Linguini with Kelp, Walnut, and Ginger Pesto, page 79

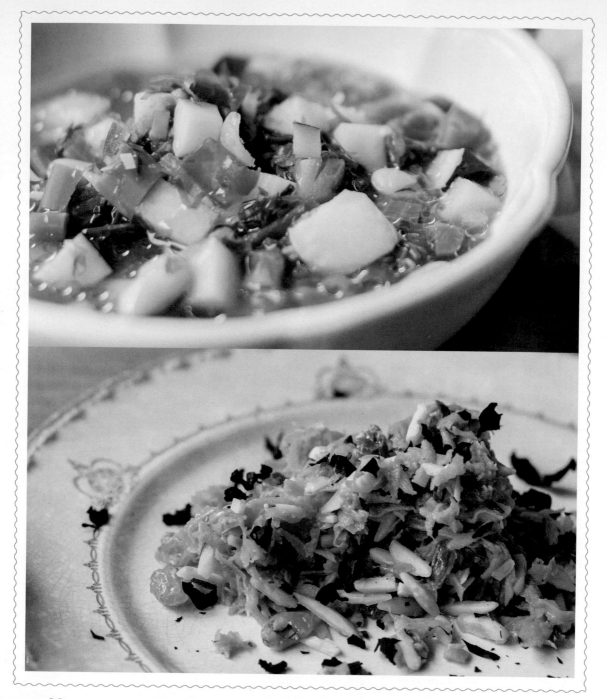

TOP: Minestrone, page 117 BOTTOM: Moroccan Salad, page 104

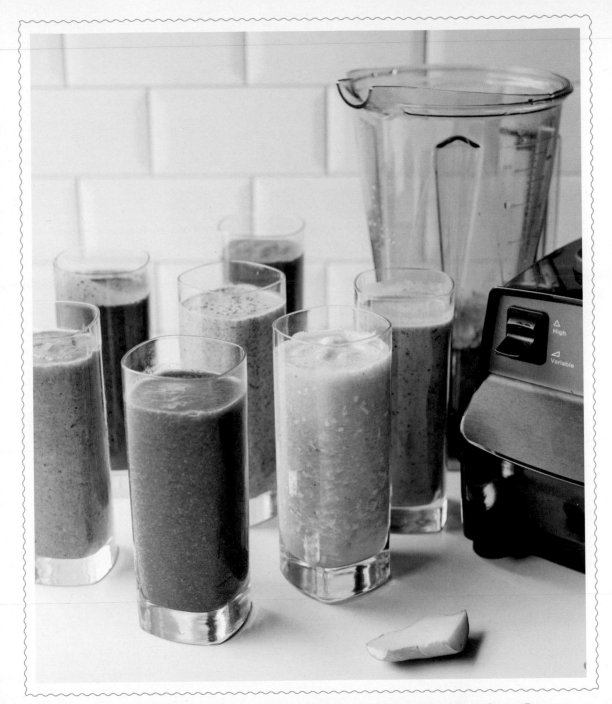

CLOCKWISE FROM FRONT CENTER: Smoothies, pages 59-61: Peach Melba, Mixed Fruit Super Green, Choco-cado, Cherry Mint, Protein Punch, Pina Colada; CENTER: Mango Margarita

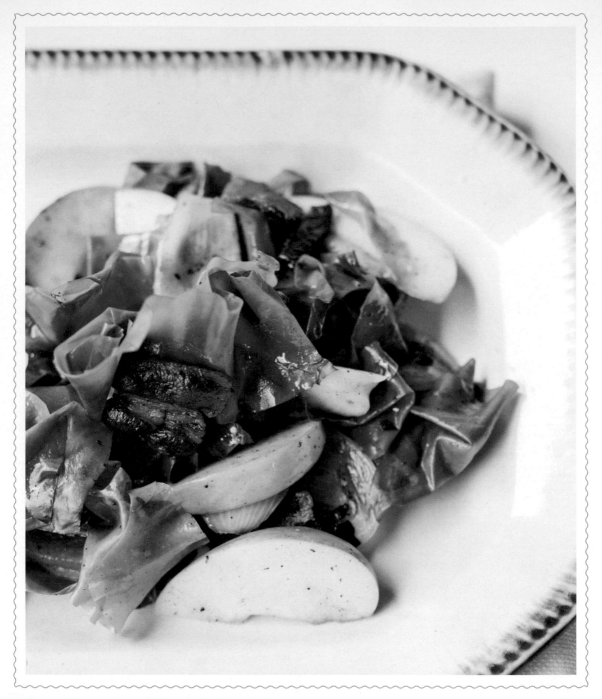

Sautéed Seagreens with Bacon, Apple, and Onion, page 91

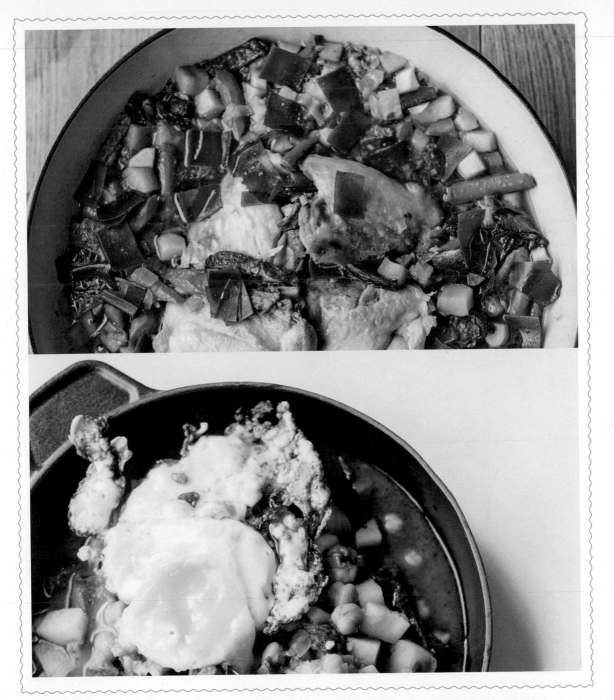

TOP: Dashi-Braised Chicken with Root Vegetables, page 125 BOTTOM: Moorish Stew, page 123

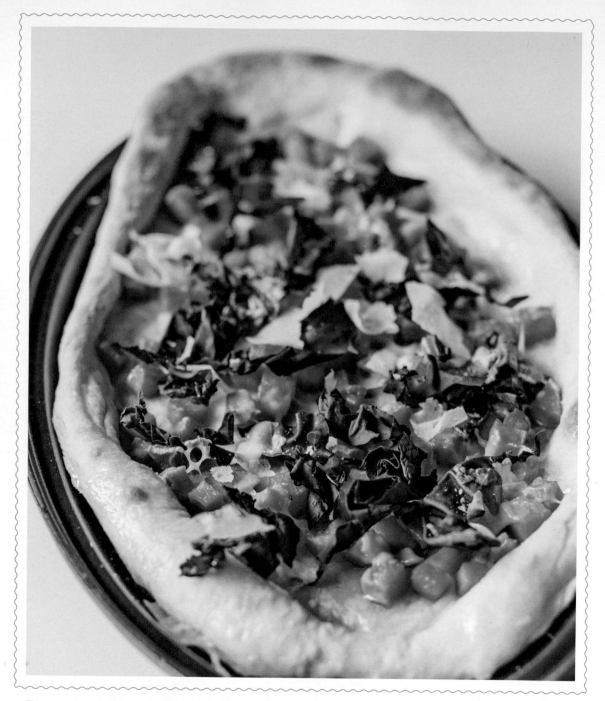

Flatbread with Butternut Squash and Smoked Dulse, page 74

IRON

Iron can be found in every cell of the human body. It is necessary for the creation of hemoglobin and myoglobin, proteins found in red blood cells and muscles, respectively. Seagreens are one of a few non-meat sources that are high in iron. Seagreens have twice as much iron and half as many calories as red meat (6 percent RDA and 110 calories in 2 ounces of grass-fed lean ground beef versus 12 percent RDA and 40 calories in 2 ounces of kelp). Other dietary iron sources include dried beans, dried fruits, eggs, liver, lean red meat, oysters, dark poultry, and salmon. For optimal iron absorption, serve seagreens with lean meat, fish, poultry, or beans, or in combination with dark leafy greens. Foods rich in vitamin C can increase iron absorption, and since seagreens have both vitamin C and iron, the iron is more bioavailable.

MAGNESIUM

Magnesium is necessary for maintaining the nervous, muscular, skeletal, and immune systems. It also aids in regulating heart rate and blood glucose levels, and it may play a role in preventing high blood pressure, heart disease, and diabetes. It's not hard to get the proper daily dose of magnesium—a

RECOMMENDED DIETARY ALLOWANCE (RDA)

For all vitamins, minerals, and nutrients, the recommended daily value per person depends on a variety of factors, including your age and gender, and whether you are pregnant, breastfeeding, or ill. For information regarding your particular recommended dietary allowance (RDA) and any dietary supplements or over-the-counter and prescription medicines you may be taking, consult your doctor, pharmacist, nutritionist/dietitian, or other health-care providers before making any change to your diet.

one-cup serving of fresh kelp contains roughly one third of the daily recommended value of magnesium.

NON-SEAGREEN SOURCES: Magnesium can also be found in dark green leafy vegetables, bananas, avocados, nuts, legumes, seeds, soy, and whole grains.

MANGANESE

Seagreens are also a good source of the nutrient manganese. Manganese is an essential nutrient required for processing cholesterol, carbohydrates, and protein. It works in conjunction with calcium and vitamin D in bone formation. Try combining seagreens with nuts, legumes, seeds, tea, whole grains, and leafy green vegetables for maximum absorption of manganese, calcium, and vitamin D.

MELATONIN

Melatonin, a hormone that regulates our sleep and wake cycles, is found in seagreens. Consuming seagreens may even help fight off jet lag and that annoying week following the change to or from daylight saving time!

PHOSPHORUS

Phosphorus is a mineral necessary for bone and teeth growth. It is also integral to metabolizing carbohydrates and fats, and in creating ATP, an energy-storing molecule. It works in conjunction with B vitamins. Phosphorus is found in every cell of the human body, although it is concentrated in the bones and teeth. Phosphorus contributes roughly 1 percent of our body weight. Dietary phosphorus is found primarily in meats and dairy products but also in vegetarian-friendly seagreens!

POLYMERS

Polymers are long chains of molecules that take on unique characteristics depending on their specific components. Studies show that red algae (such as dulse, carrageenan, and laver), which contain the polymers agar and carrageenan, are an effective respiratory treatment. In fact, carrageenan has been used for centuries to treat respiratory ailments such as sinus infections, pneumonia, and asthma (the Maya prepared a thick, restorative beverage made with a carrageenan-thickened liquid composed of ground cacao, vanilla bean, and honey). Carrageenans also appear to have antiviral properties.

PHYCOPOLYMERS

Seaweeds are generally divided into green, red, and brown algae. Seaweeds are made up of 25–40 percent mucopolysaccharides, which are collectively referred to as phycopolymers. The

ALGINATES AND HEAVY METAL PROTECTION

Alginates help prevent the absorption of mercury, cadmium, plutonium, cesium, and other toxic metals. For example, sodium alginate in kelp protects the body against radiation absorption, specifically strontium 90, a by-product of nuclear facilities.

brown algal phycopolymers are alginic acid (also called algin or alginate) and fucoidan.

Algin has unique thickening properties that are used in a variety of ways. It can be used for medicinal purposes, for example, to lower cholesterol, to reduce heavy metals in the body, or to treat and prevent high blood pressure. Sodium alginate is a naturally occurring polysaccharide found in brown seaweeds and is used as a thickener in many dairy products. A handy ingredient in the kitchen, algin has gelling qualities that do not require heat, and it can be used to give food products a rich, silky-smooth texture. Algin can also be used as a binding agent in pills and capsules—you've probably taken it in gel caps!

Fucoidan, the other algal phycopolymer found in various species of brown algae, is used in some dietary supplements. It has also been shown to have anticoagulant and antiviral properties, and it may even help prevent the growth of cancer cells.

POTASSIUM

Potassium, a mineral found in seagreens, is essential to muscle function, building proteins, regulating body pH levels, and controlling the electrical activity of the heart. Given that seagreens are grown in a saltwater environment, naturally they have a higher salt content than foods grown in soil. The salt in seagreens also has a different makeup than cooking or table salt (NaCl), which has increasingly been shown to have negative effects on our health—largely due to overconsumption.

However, because there is more potassium in the salt found in seagreens, it reacts differently with the body, and it has been shown to not have the adverse effects of NaCl. Yet seagreen salt can be used to season foods in the same satisfying way as table salt. If you are looking to reduce your intake of sodium, flaked or powdered seagreens are a great alternative.

NON-SEAGREEN SOURCES: Red meats and fish, soy, broccoli, peas, lima beans, tomatoes, potatoes, sweet potatoes, winter squash, citrus fruits, cantaloupe, bananas, kiwi, prunes, apricots, dairy products, and nuts.

People with kidney (renal) ailments should limit consumption of potassium-rich foods. Consult your doctor before introducing seagreens into your diet.

If you're like most people I know, you've tried a protein shake or two as a way to boost your recovery after a workout. Commercial protein powders made from whey, soy, and casein are the most common, particularly whey. But experts disagree on the efficacy of protein powders. The prevalent opinion is that although they may be easy and convenient, they are most likely unnecessary, and frequently their high calorie count is not worth the extra nutrition. In fact, protein shakes are generally not recommended as a post-workout beverage. To rebuild and fuel muscle cells, the body needs a ratio of four to five grams of protein to one gram of carbohydrate. Most protein powders contain at least twenty grams of protein per serving, which would require eighty grams of carbohydrates to balance the nutrient proportion. With all the nutrients in seagreens, including vitamins, minerals, protein, and electrolytes, a better post-workout protein drink would be a seagreens smoothie. Made with yogurt or milk, these smoothies have everything your body needs for a speedy recovery after a hard workout—try Cherry Mint Smoothie on page 60.

PROTEIN

Proteins, referred to as the building blocks of life, are macronutrients that create and repair cells comprised of amino acid chains. As proteins are digested, they are broken down into amino acids. Amino acids are classified as essential, nonessential, and conditional.

- ESSENTIAL AMINO ACIDS cannot be created by the body and must be consumed via diet. Essential amino acids can be eaten together or separately over the course of a day. Balance of amino acid consumption in the diet is important to ensure complete protein absorption.

- NONESSENTIAL AMINO ACIDS can be made by the body by breaking down essential amino acids.

- CONDITIONAL AMINO ACIDS are not necessary for daily bodily function but are necessary in combating illness and stress.

Seagreens contain more than twenty different amino acids and have a combined amino acid score of seventy-nine out of one hundred, meaning that seagreens are a good source of several amino acids—most importantly, histidine. To ensure complete protein consumption, combine seagreens with foods such as bananas and chia seeds, which have high histidine-to-tryptophan ratios.

The protein quantity in seagreens is not sufficient to be the only form of protein you take in, but all the essential amino acids can be found in most types of seagreens. You don't have to eat red meat in order to get all the protein your body needs. Eating a variety of plant proteins can provide ample dietary protein. Combining them with other incomplete plant proteins will augment the amino acids and provide plenty of vegan protein.

NON-MEAT COMPLETE PROTEINS INCLUDE: Quinoa (8 grams/cup), buckwheat (6 grams/cup), hempseed (10 grams/2 tablespoons), chia seeds (4 grams/2 tablespoons), and soy products (10 grams/½ cup firm tofu).

COMPLETE VERSUS INCOMPLETE PROTEINS

Complete proteins contain all nine essential amino acids. These are generally found in animal products. Incomplete proteins may be missing one or more of the essential amino acids. Seagreens have trace amounts of all amino acids but are not sufficient to be the only form of protein in the diet. Try serving them with other complete or incomplete protein items to provide proper dietary protein.

EAT THE WHOLE THING

As with most foods, the whole food offers more complete nutrition than when it is broken down into its components. Seagreens in pill form, as a supplement, may contain a quantity of vitamins and minerals in levels that may have an unpredictable impact on your health. Check with a nutritionist or your doctor to learn more about dietary supplements.

SELENIUM

Selenium aids in many systems, including the reproductive and immune systems, the thyroid, and DNA production. It is a mineral found in soil and water that is absorbed by plants and animals as they grow. The mineral-rich waters where seagreens grow give them plenty of selenium. Many studies suggest that people who consume lower amounts of selenium may have an increased risk of a host of ailments and diseases ranging from cancer to heart disease and thyroid disease. Blood selenium levels decrease with age, and this may be linked to decreased brain function.

NON-SEAGREEN SOURCES: Mushrooms, legumes, seeds, nuts, grains, rice, broccoli, cabbage, and spinach.

SODIUM

We need sodium for proper nerve function and to balance the water and mineral content in our bodies. However, too much sodium—too much salt in our diet—can cause a host of ailments, including high blood pressure, heart disease, and stroke. Seagreens contain less than 5 percent of the RDA of sodium per cup and impart a salty flavor to food without increasing the sodium content (at least not by much), making them both tasty and heart healthy.

STEROLS

Phytochemicals are chemicals found in plants. Plant sterols are phytochemicals that may lower blood cholesterol by blocking the absorption of cholesterol in the small intestine. Seagreens contain these cholesterol-blocking sterols.

ELECTROLYTES

Electrolytes are more than just a mysterious ingredient found in neon-colored sports beverages. Electrolytes are naturally found in your body. They control the pH of your blood and the water levels in your body. Electrolytes can come in the form of acids, bases, and salts. When you sweat, you lose electrolytes. They must be replaced by electrolyte-containing fluids; water alone will not replace them. Luckily for us, seagreens contain several different electrolytes, such as calcium, magnesium, phosphorus, and potassium, and can aid in rehydration.

OMEGA FATTY ACIDS

Seagreens contain healthy omega-3 fatty acids. These are polyunsaturated fatty acid chains. There are various forms of omega-3s—EPA, DHA, and ALA are three of the most common ones. EPA and DHA are found in seafood and shellfish. ALA can be found in other plant-based foods, including flaxseeds, and canola and soy oils, as well as some seagreens. Evidence suggests that omega-3 consumption can decrease risk of heart disease. Omega-3s are also critical to fetal growth and development and may have positive results in alleviating symptoms of rheumatoid arthritis as well as contributing to healthy brain and eye function.

Omega-6 fatty acids are also considered essential fatty acids. The body cannot make

WHERE THE CALORIES COME FROM

The calories in seagreens come mostly from carbohydrates (79 percent). Fats (11 percent) and protein (10 percent) make up the rest.

omega fatty acids on its own and must absorb them from food sources. Omega-6 fatty acids, along with omega-3s, are critical for brain function, growth, and development. For optimal health, experts recommend a balance of omega-3s and omega-6s in the one-to-one to one-to-two range. The typical American diet, however, contains fourteen to twenty-five times more omega-6 fatty acids than omega-3 fatty acids. Eating seagreens can help shift the balance! Studies have shown omega-6 fatty acids, when balanced with omega-3 fatty acids, can have positive effects on diabetic neuropathy, rheumatoid arthritis, allergies, attention-deficit/hyperactivity disorder (ADHD), breast cancer treatments, eczema, and high blood pressure (hypertension), among others.

FIBER

Seagreens are high in dietary fiber. A cup of fresh kelp has more than 30 percent of the RDA of dietary fiber. It aids in digestion, lowers LDL (bad) cholesterol levels, and helps control blood sugar levels.

A carboyhdrate, fiber may be listed as soluable fiber or insoluable fiber on nutritional labels. Both types are important to human health—and both are found in seagreens.

- SOLUBLE FIBER dissolves in water and forms a gel-like substance that may help

> **DID YOU KNOW?**
>
> Kelp may improve the balance and functioning of intestinal flora. It also has properties that expel intestinal worms.

lower blood glucose and cholesterol levels. It is found in oats, peas, beans, apples, and citrus fruits.

- INSOLUBLE FIBER does not dissolve in water and passes through the digestive tract, providing stool bulk. It is found in whole grains, nuts, legumes, and many vegetables.

If you're concerned with weight loss, fiber can make you feel full faster, eat less, and lose weight. Fiber isn't digested by your body; instead, it passes through the digestive tract, aiding digestion and preventing constipation. At least one study indicates that breads made with high-fiber seagreens can aid in weight loss. Hours after eating bread baked with seagreens, participants reported feeling full and ate significantly less at the next meal.

Consuming too much fiber at once however, can cause intestinal discomfort. Be sure to drink plenty of water, as fiber works best when it absorbs water. Don't make any dietary changes too quickly—introduce a small amount of a new food at a time—and always consult with your health-care professional beforehand.

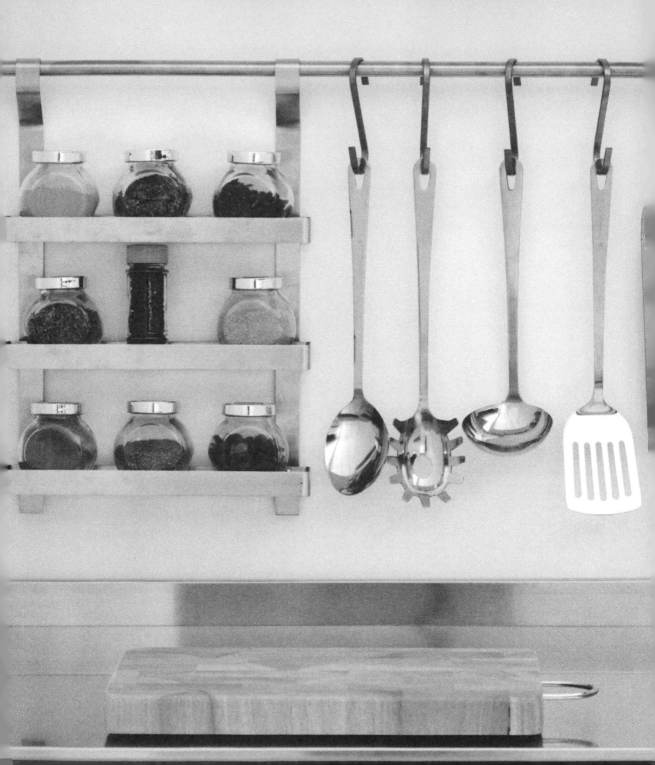

CHAPTER 4

EQUIPPING YOUR KITCHEN AND PANTRY

One of the true keys to a successful dinner is to have a great plan of action before you start. The best way to accomplish this is to have all of your ingredients in front of you—in the order you'll need them—before you begin cooking. If your ingredients are all over the kitchen, you will be, too. Dinner is about enjoying your family and company, about relaxing and attending to the easy alchemy of delicious ingredients coming together. So bring the process into focus before your attention wanders.

TOOLS

While a good craftsman never blames his or her tools, a good craftsman knows it really helps to have great tools. Although it is true that many of the recommended items below require some investment, they return even greater value. Not only do they last as long as you take care of them (sometimes for generations), they can help to make you a better cook through one simple benefit: consistency. When you use just a few tools and really get to know them and how they behave, then you have reduced a great variable in the practice of cooking. When a tool becomes familiar, it allows you to cook more fluently, so that you can focus on the ingredients and less on the mechanics.

- CUTTING BOARD. Many of your ingredients have to pass over your cutting board, so why not just keep what you need right there, within easy reach. In my kitchen, other than my knife, there is no tool as essential as my giant cutting board. It allows me to organize as I work, arranging ingredients in the order they will be used, and still have plenty of space in which to chop whatever comes next. Making the investment in a big, high-quality wood board, such as a Boos Block™, is well worth it—not only does it make cooking more efficient and enjoyable, it's also a beautiful addition to your kitchen.

- BLENDER. Many of the recipes in this book call for seagreens to be used in a purée, whether as a pesto, gazpacho, or smoothie. Having a great blender makes all the difference in the world. In fact, I've found that a good blender is an essential tool that has helped me stay committed to healthier breakfast choices. I made the investment in a Vitamix™ blender and have never once regretted it. It has lasted me for more than a decade and is the key to my morning routine. The powerful motor can turn frozen fruit, seagreens, and any challenge I throw at into a beautiful purée.

Even better, the cleanup is easy. After pouring out my smoothie, I add a few drops of soap and a bit of water into the canister and blend until it's clean. Simply rinse it off and you're done. Why do I mention this? Because good habits are easy to start but are much harder to keep. If the task is simple, I find that I am far more likely to stick with it. Drinking a less-than-smooth smoothie or coming home to a dirty blender caked with dried smoothie is a real turnoff. When the task is made easy by using the proper equipment, you might find you have a bit more resolve in achieving your goals.

Oh, and the Vitamix makes a mean margarita when you blend tequila and triple sec with a touch of frozen fruit for a nontraditional but refreshing potion.

HERE ARE SOME OF MY GO-TO ESSENTIALS

- **A SET OF J. A. HENCKELS™ NONSTICK SAUTÉ PANS.** This heavy-bottomed cookware heats quickly and holds a remarkably constant temperature, which takes a lot of the guesswork out of cooking. Plus, the nonstick coating is really nonstick. After cooking, just give whatever pan you've used a quick wipe with some paper towels and it's ready to go again. Although a gentle rinse with a nonabrasive sponge or cloth is recommended from time to time, these pans require little maintenance, but they must be handled with care in order to maintain the integrity of the surface.

- **HEAT-PROOF RUBBER SPATULAS.** Get four or five of these and always have them within reach. Not only are they forgiving if exposed to heat, they are as gentle on high-quality pans as a tool should be.

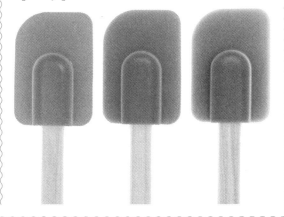

- **FAVORITE KNIVES.** Most cooks don't need more than a few knives. In my kitchen J. A. Henckels knives fit the bill, as they are easy to sharpen, incredibly durable, and beautifully designed. A paring knife, a six-inch chef's or utility knife, a ten-inch chef's knife, and a serrated bread knife will accomplish almost any task faced by the home cook.

- **JAPANESE MANDOLINE.** This is an essential tool found in every professional kitchen. The plastic board fitted with a centered razor blade makes prepping vegetables an easy task and yields an impressively perfect cut. This is the tool for making paper-thin slices of radish, onion, fennel, and any other crunchy vegetable you can think of. Additional attachments can easily be added to turn vegetables like carrots into thin strands, wisps of texture perfect for stir-fries and salads. The only caveat is that more than almost any other kitchen tool, the mandoline must be used with the utmost attention and caution because it does not know the difference between a carrot and a finger. Just as with any other tool, attention to detail is key.

- **STAUB™ COCOTTES.** This heavy-bottomed enameled cast-iron cookware is the workhorse in my kitchen. I have a number of these pans, ranging from four quarts and up, and I use them for everything from boiling vegetables to making stocks, sauces, soups, and braised dishes.

- **A GOOD PEPPER GRINDER.** Preground pepper, ground lord knows when, is a bit of an assault on the foods you've just lovingly prepared—lost are all the heady floral perfumes and the fresh, sharp bite of freshly ground pepper, one of the most charismatic ingredients in cooking. A quality pepper mill, adjustable to allow for varying sizes of ground pepper, on the other hand, gives this superb ingredient a chance to shine when freshly ground over food just as you serve it.

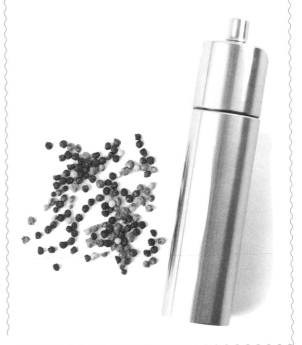

MY PERFECT PANTRY

Having a well-stocked pantry can boil down to a lot of inventory, but here's my argument for fully stocked cupboards: more often than not, good food happens by virtue of good ingredients that are accentuated by relatively simply means. A salad of good peppery greens, enlivened by just the right vinegar, results in the perfect balance of sweet and tang, and a perfectly good sandwich can become that much better with the addition of just the right whole grain mustard. Now, you don't need to go overboard: you don't need ten different kinds of mustard. But having a pantry of go-to ingredients allows you to enjoy every meal that much more. And most pantry items have a very long shelf life, so while there may be an initial investment, products won't go to waste, and you'll reap the benefits of more enjoyable meals for a long time to come.

Here are a few great staples to keep on hand:

• **VINEGARS.** Have several of these on hand, including good-quality white and red wine vinegars, balsamic vinegar, and my favorite, sherry vinegar. The addition of vinegar, a very complex and elegant acid, will highlight and accent the natural flavors of almost any dish.

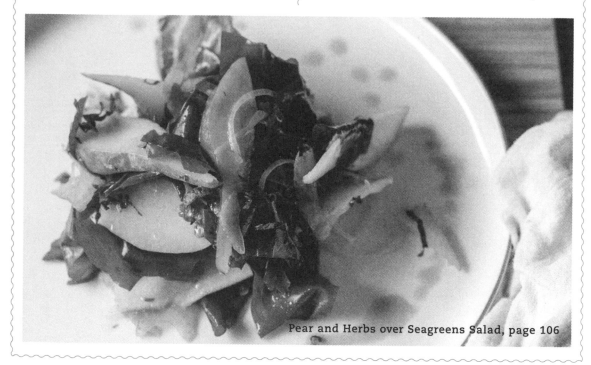

Pear and Herbs over Seagreens Salad, page 106

- OLIVE OIL. Find a brand you really like, preferably a mild, extra virgin oil—it will bring beauty and finesse to any dish—and buy it in bulk (don't be afraid to use a lot).

- HOT SAUCE. The acidic bite of Tabasco™ or Crystal™ always finds favor when you add it to a dish. I also like some of the purée-style hot sauces, such as Tapatio™, which have a little more complexity and depth to them, and bring floral and fruity notes to a dish along with the heat.

- MIRIN. This sweetened rice cooking wine has a beautiful aroma of lemon blossoms and honey. Mild in its sweetness, it brings balance to dishes with a spike of acid. Try it with more earthy ingredients like lentils or buckwheat noodles, too.

- SESAME OIL. I always use toasted sesame oil, as the flavors are so nicely developed. Buy it in small quantities because a little goes a long way, and it can go off if it is not used within a few months.

- NUT OILS. Whether it's walnut, almond, or pistachio oil, nut oils bring their wonderful aroma and flavor to a dish without adding texture. A little bit goes a long way.

- BROWN RICE. Although it takes longer to cook than its white counterpart, the nutritive value of brown rice is significantly higher. It also has a robust nutty flavor, adding both nutritional value and interest to any meal.

- QUINOA. This staple crop of South America has made its way into North America's shopping aisles as well as our hearts. Quinoa is a complete protein, making it a favorite among vegetarians and healthy eaters. A tip on preparation: quinoa should always be washed under cold running water for three to five minutes prior to cooking. This removes any traces of the bitter powder that covers the outside.

- BARLEY. Barley is a wonderfully versatile grain. Whether it's cooked in soups and stews or mixed with fresh ingredients to make a quick salad, barley is prized for its snappy texture and nutty flavor.

- WHOLE WHEAT PASTA. Whole wheat pasta adds nutrition to a staple dish that has become a regular weeknight meal for lots of folks. Its brown color indicates a nutty flavor, the perfect foil for vegetable-laden pasta dishes.

- NUTS. I keep a wide variety of nuts on hand at all times. Adding them to almost any dish delivers a quick, delicious, nutritious crunch. Whether they are toasted or enjoyed raw, nuts add a wonderful complexity and sometimes an unexpected twist to everyday dishes.

- **GOLDEN RAISINS.** Sweeter and plumper than their dark cousins, golden raisins are completely interchangeable with regular dark raisins; however, I feel they have a better appearance on the plate. Try giving them a quick soak in vinegar and water before adding them to salads or vegetable dishes.

- **WHOLE GRAIN MUSTARD.** The snappy bite of little mustard seeds and the tang of vinegar make whole grain mustard a very elegant (and delicious) ingredient, especially when it's added to salad dressings. It makes for a visually appealing component to a salad as well.

- **DIJON MUSTARD.** Perfect for whisking into vinaigrettes to make creamy-style dressings without unwanted dairy or calories, the potent flavor of Dijon mustard lends its spark to the personality of any dish through its slight lingering spice.

- **WORCESTERSHIRE SAUCE.** Dark and brooding, this familiar (and yet tough to spell) sauce is a mixture of many different sweet, sour, and aromatic ingredients and lends instant depth and interest to any dish it is used in.

- **SARDINES AND ANCHOVIES (CANNED).** Using a few sardines or anchovies is the perfect way to add nutrition to any dish from salad dressings to vegetable sautés. Even people who don't love them on their own often find sardines and anchovies to be delightful when they are included in a dish as a flavoring. Make sure to use the oil they are packed in, as it has a wonderful flavor and plenty of nutrition as well.

- **FIRE-ROASTED DICED TOMATOES (CANNED).** These tomatoes are one of the most convenient go-to ingredients to have on hand, as they bring great color, flavor, and freshness to dishes. I prefer to use fire-roasted tomatoes, as they have less of the acid taste of raw tomatoes, making them perfect for last-minute additions.

- **CORNMEAL.** Too often we think of this ingredient as a product that can be kept in the pantry year-round without losing its freshness or flavor, but even humble cornmeal has its season. Look for freshly milled products, such as Bob's Red Mill™. The resulting dish will be so much more flavorful and compelling!

- **BEANS (CANNED).** Beans are incredibly economical, convenient, and nutritious—and you can jazz them up with a host of delicious flavors while they're cooking. Before using them, be sure to wash and drain them to remove the starchy canning liquid. Canned beans can be very salty, so be sure to keep that in mind before adding salt to a dish.

- **SPICES AND DRIED HERBS.** In nearly all dishes I prefer the ebullient, bright flavor of fresh herbs to that of dried herbs; however, dried herbs offer a charismatic personality all their own. When they're added to winter dishes, dried herbs can remind us of warm days ahead. I also rely heavily on spices to provide depth and character to my meals. A lot of cooks make the mistake of segregating spices between baking and savory applications. But traditional baking spices such as star anise, allspice, and nutmeg are all equally, if not more, interesting when they're used in savory dishes.

- **CHILE PEPPERS.** Chile peppers, in various degrees of heat, add complexity to food through their floral and fruity flavors. I keep a range of whole, flaked, and powdered chiles on hand. I add whole chiles to dishes, simmering them into sauces and stews, and use chile powders and flakes as I would black pepper to season dishes.

- **KOSHER SALT.** There are so many options for salt out there, it's hard to know which one to use. My rule of thumb is to use just one. Different salts have various levels of salinity by volume, making them as tricky to use as any other unfamiliar seasoning, so I use kosher salt because I know how it will perform every time I use it. Feel free to use any salt you like, but use just one and get good at using it.

- **GINGER AND GARLIC.** Both of these ingredients can be simmered into oil or butter at the beginning of the cooking process, which carries their aromatic flavors throughout the dish. Grated or whole, garlic is usually left in a dish, whereas ginger is removed, more often than not, unless it has been grated.

- **LEMONS AND LIMES.** These lovely citrus fruits help to bring balance to dishes by adding their sweet/bitter personality along with their floral aroma. I find that lime pairs best with many fresh herbs, and lemon supplies the perfect finishing jolt to cooked dishes such as beef stew and seafood pasta.

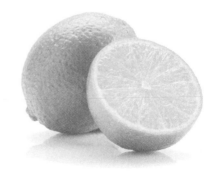

SEAGREEN-FRIENDLY HERBS

Culinary herbs are an incredible way to add flavor, personality, and nutrition to dishes. Unfortunately, herbs are too often relegated to playing only the role of a garnish, an afterthought, added just for appearances. But the flavors of herbs are among the most valuable in many kitchens (in mine, certainly). Their clarity and ebullience are something to showcase, not use just as a sprinkling at the end. Large handfuls of herbs, for example, bring incredible complexity to salads, which can otherwise be rather pedestrian dishes. When sautéing or steaming vegetables, such as broccoli scented with a bit of olive oil, toss in a big handful of freshly chopped herbs right at the end to provide a vibrancy that might actually get your kids to eat these greens.

Herbs can have very different personalities. I characterize them as "hard" or "soft." Hard herbs, like rosemary, thyme, oregano, lavender, and bay leaf, are best when added at the beginning of the cooking process, so that their powerful personalities and bold accent have time to soften and integrate into dishes. Usually, these herbs are removed prior to serving, as their flavor is apparent without a physical presence. Soft herbs are far more delicate in their properties, texture, flavor, and strength than hard herbs, and they are usually added at the end of cooking. Their volatile oils are best flattered when gently warmed by other components in a dish. Their aromas generally provide a bit of levity, with their fresh and delightful perfume, to foods such as zucchini or seagreens, whose flavors might have become slightly muted during cooking. The vibrancy of fresh herbs cannot be understated.

BASIL

No list of herbs would be complete without mention of basil. However, to my taste, basil simply does not pair well with many seagreens. Its floral and soaringly aromatic character simply does not flatter the briny personality of seagreens.

BAY LEAF

Bay leaf is commonly used both fresh and dry. The leaf of a laurel bush or tree commonly found in areas with a Mediterranean climate, it has a very distinct personality when fresh and a more nuanced flavor when dry, lending depth and structure to whatever it is added to. In either form, it is always added to liquids, where its essential oils are extracted and carried through a dish via the broth. The texture of the leaf is not palatable, however, and it should be removed before serving. Especially when fresh, bay leaf has a rather

In my opinion, fresh herbs are best used to finish a dish with their clean, fresh flavors. Dried herbs, which are bolder in character, are better used sparingly when at the beginning of the cooking process. While dried and fresh herbs are often interchangeable, the only herb I prefer in the dried form is oregano. When raw, this herb can be very brash, and it is too distinct for most applications. The dried version has a much mellower personality and is much friendlier with accompanying ingredients.

eucalyptus-like scent, which some people find is reminiscent of soap. With seagreens, bay leaf is best when it is paired with the bolder flavors of dulse or sea lettuce.

CHERVIL

Chervil is the softest of the "soft" herbs. Its incredibly delicate, lacy, silken texture gets lost in many preparations. To me, its best use is as a flowery flourish to be added to cold dishes seconds before serving. The incredibly delicate anise- and lemon-like scent of chervil, though very reserved, can make a huge impact. Paired with seagreens, chervil can make a nice textural contrast to crunchy dried wakame and add a little bit of volume to a more traditional seagreen salad flavored in the Asian tradition. Chervil pairs particularly well with the subtle punch of chile flakes.

CILANTRO

Although cilantro is widely considered a Tex-Mex ingredient, its range of culinary application extends far beyond the Southwest to Asian, African, and northern European cuisines. Also called Chinese parsley, cilantro is very enigmatic in that it can bring warmth and charm to seagreen preparations such as dashi or salads made of rehydrated dulse. It can also have incredible cooling properties when it is chopped fresh and added to long-simmered vegetable dishes, such as seagreens and beans, just prior to serving. The strong flavor of cilantro can be off-putting to some people who perceive the flavor as soapy. This affects only a portion of the population, however, and the genetic science as to why this happens is somewhat complicated.

DILL

Dill is best characterized as a "cool" herb. The feathery, frill-like fronds are exceedingly delicate in texture and their flavor is deceptively strong, not in its assertiveness but rather in its ability to weave its personality seamlessly in a dish, even in small quantities. Dill can really accentuate the cold nature of seagreens—not always a flattering pairing. On the other hand, dill works beautifully with seagreens when they're combined with a fruit, particularly an aromatic one, such as apple, pear, or fresh plum.

GREEN ONIONS (SCALLIONS)

While some may argue over whether the green onion is a vegetable or an herb, I put it in the herb category because of the way I use it in my cooking. A green onion has two different personalities: the top has the soft texture and sweetness of a spring green, and the bottom, the white bulb, by contrast, has a delicate, sharp crunch. Green onions differ from traditional onions in that they are softer in texture, making them far easier to integrate into dishes. And where other onions can be used raw or cooked, green onions are really best used as a finishing ingredient. When tossed into soups or broths, green onions maintain their gentle crunch; when they are added to salads, their texture is a nice accent to lighter, leafier greens. And because they are not overly spicy, green onions' whisper of piquancy brings a bit of balance to dishes that include chiles.

OREGANO (DRIED)

When paired with olive oil, the flavor of dried oregano is allowed to soften. Mellowing through the richness of the oil, it can provide a very interesting platform for the saltiness of seagreens. While so many ingredients are global in their flavors and applications, oregano always strikes me as a purely Mediterranean ingredient. When paired with seagreens, it recalls the potent, warm, sweet breezes of that romantic clime.

PARSLEY

To my mind parsley is only useful in its flat-leaf form. The curly parsley commonly used in Middle Eastern cuisines can be too grassy and taste too overpoweringly green for my kitchen. The flat-leaf variety offers a svelte or gentlemanly personality that, while it is certainly noticeable in any dish in which it is included, also makes a great dance partner for many other ingredients. With seagreens, flat-leaf parsley is particularly amenable as a partner in pesto recipes and as a finishing perfume to dashi broths and restorative teas. In dishes such as a quiche or frittata, where the seagreens' color can become less handsome during the cooking process, the visually appealing green fleck of parsley can save the day.

CHOPPING FRESH HERBS

Not only are fresh herbs often neglected as an opportunity to enliven cooking, they are all too often abused before ever seeing a plate. The first key is to buy the freshest herbs you can find. (Snipping them fresh from your kitchen garden can't be beat.) The next key is to use an exceedingly sharp knife: the essential oils that are so coveted in fresh herbs can be lost due to overoxidation brought on by bruising and mishandling. Those fancy chefs you see hacking away at herbs with two knives at a time, bits flying about, are impressive for sure, but to my mind, these folks don't really know what they're doing.

To chop fresh herbs, take a quantity and arrange them neatly, slightly rolling them together so that the leaves and stems are relatively compact. Hold the herbs together tightly, without bruising them; then use a sharp knife to slice across the arrangement of herbs. You are not pressing down so much as slicing through them. As you cut down the stems, continually rearrange them with your fingers to keep them in a tight bundle. Do not move the herbs, but rather move yourself or the cutting board, so you may repeat the same slicing process in the opposite direction, slicing crosswise against the first slices of herbs you made. In this way, the herbs will be sliced with the minimal possible contact. Without any extra pounding or chopping, you end up with the clearest, cleanest flavor, and you also retain the beautiful brilliant green color of the herbs. Yes, the pieces may not be completely uniform and even, but uniform and even is not the purpose of cooking. Delicious is the purpose.

TARRAGON

Tarragon has the personality of the wizened and confident old professor, humbled nonetheless to work with less distinguished peers to create delicious dishes. Tarragon is best when chopped fresh as a final addition to a dish, especially salads. A little bit goes a very long way, so judicious use is recommended. Tarragon can also be steeped into broths or soups to lend elegance and a charismatic touch.

THYME

This "hard" herb, in its many forms, lends an earthy base layer of flavor to dishes, bringing both surf and turf flavors into play. When it is paired with the iodine tang of seagreens, the flavor of thyme can take on a somewhat cardboard flavor. However, freshly chopped and paired with rehydrated seagreens, its personality can be coaxed out in a simple dressing of red wine vinegar, grated garlic, and extra virgin olive oil plus cool ingredients, such as tomato and cucumber.

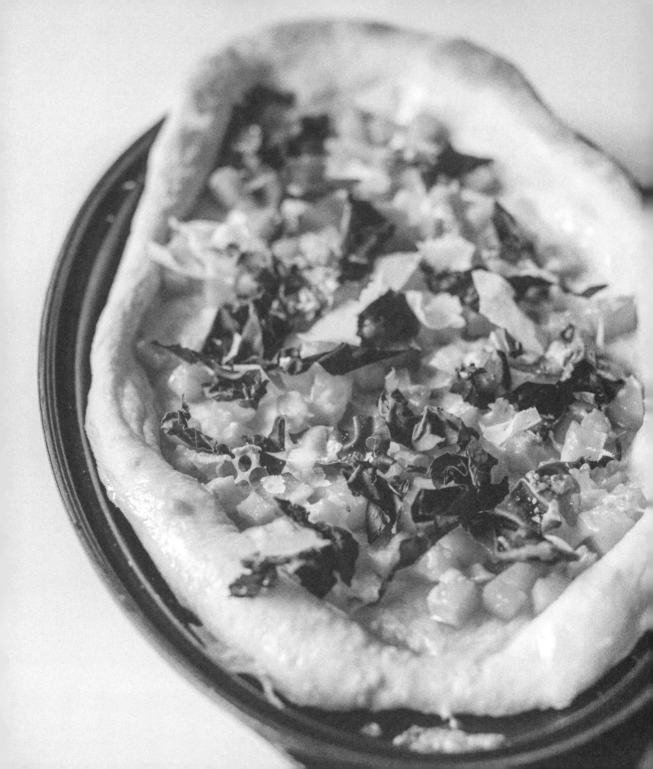

CHAPTER 5

BUYING AND PREPARING SEAGREENS

For those of you who are unfamiliar with seagreens, this unique, versatile, and delicious resource gives you the opportunity to incorporate more greens—of all kinds—into your diet. And, because we are constantly urged to increase our consumption of vegetables and eat less meat, more and more people are turning to the vegetable and bulk food aisles for a larger portion of their dinner plate. This hopeful trend has led to the incredible rise in popularity of various products—for example, the meteoric ascension of kale, a phenomenon unlike any other I have witnessed. As the general quality of produce has improved, along with our popular interests, the variety of produce and related products has risen accordingly. We currently have access in many stores to five or six varieties of chile pepper; ten different kinds of salad greens; purple, cheddar, and traditional white cauliflowers; a dozen types of apples—you name it, diversity is everywhere. And that's a good thing. With our tastes shifting toward plant-based foods, I urge you to begin thinking even beyond the produce aisle for regular sustenance, variety, and a palette of fresh new flavors.

The uses and nutritional properties of seagreens as a culinary ingredient are similar to if not the same as many ingredients already in your repertoire. Given that seagreens have an exciting and unique flavor profile, some folks will take to them immediately, while others might need a more gentle entry. For those who love them, seagreens make an excellent centerpiece to a meal or a memorable side dish. For those who seek a softer landing, seagreens can be incorporated into some foods or used to replace a portion of more familiar ingredients, such as in Zucchini-Seagreen Bread (see page 137) or smoothies (see pages 55–61). The recipes in this book employ both methods of introduction. For instance, a simple seagreens sauté is an acknowledgment of our familiarity with spinach and kale, torn leaves scattered over a flatbread give a nod to the universal popularity of pizza, and smoothie recipes incorporate a wide variety of convenient fresh and frozen fruits and vegetables (cherries, blueberries, wheatgrass juice, you name it) that hopefully already have a place in your fridge or freezer. Opportunities to use these deeply flavorful, colorful ingredients are endless and lend an easy hand to the welcome of seagreens. Seagreens and their characteristic umami-rich flavors (see page 14) also make for wonderful additions to seasoning mixes for use on grilled steak or chicken, broiled fish, or seafood boils. Try mixing some dulse flakes into an Old Bay–style seasoning or bring the salty tang of sea lettuce to Herbes de Provence—all incredible and flattering ways to introduce an excitingly new, delicious, and nutritious food.

BUYING SEAGREENS

Seagreens are available in many market forms—dried, frozen, and, increasingly, fresh—and can be found at the seafood counter, in the frozen case, and in bulk food aisles of many traditional supermarkets. Please do not be put off by thinking seagreens are available only in places you don't usually shop.

Once you start looking for them, you'll find them everywhere, from your local health food store to Whole Foods Market™ to big-box grocery stores. If you can't find the one you're looking for, ask your local store to stock it, or order it online.

The recipes in this book are designed to be flexible in terms of fresh seagreens and seagreen products (usually dried or processed in some other way) that can be used. In most cases, any available variety of seagreen will work in any recipe. The exception is when making a salad, where the volume of a fresh product is needed and cannot be adequately replaced with dried seagreens. As you substitute ingredients, be aware that dried products are far more intense in flavor than fresh items, and powdered seagreens are even stronger in flavor. Be brave with substitutions, but the best advice is to add just a little at a time, until the flavor is to your liking.

One of my favorite brands is sold nationally, as well as online: Maine Coast Sea Vegetables (www.seaveg.com/shop). They specialize in sustainably harvested seagreens from the North Atlantic, offering dulse, kelp, alaria, laver, sea lettuce, bladderwrack, rockweed, and Irish moss. Their freshly harvested sea vegetables are low-temperature dried and hand packed with minimal processing at their facility in Maine. They are certified organic, gluten-free, soy-free, dairy-free, and GMO-free.

Seaweed Iceland™ products, including kombu, wakame, and dulse, are widely available at both health food stores and online retailers. The company, based in Iceland, hand harvests wild seaweed in a sustainable manner and uses renewable geothermal heat in their cold-drying process.

I have also enjoyed Emerald Cove™ dried products, which can be found in grocery stores nationally, as well as through online retailers. They sell a variety of Pacific-grown, often organic, varieties of seagreens, including nori sheets, wakame, arame, and kombu.

For seagreen powder, I use Hoosier Hill Farm's™ icelandic kelp powder (www.hoosierhillfarm.com).

You can also find seagreen products at your local Asian market. Try to find brands that are labeled with the name of the species and have been tested for heavy metals and contamination. Kelp varieties are the best bet. Avoid hijiki of unknown provenance, as it may contain high levels of toxins.

FRESH SEAGREENS

You can harvest your own seagreens, depending on your location and the time of year. Contact your local Sea Grant or Department of Natural Resources branch for guidelines and regulations for harvesting seagreens in your area. Better yet, find a seagreen farmer—perhaps at your local farmers' market—to stock up. And of course you can ask your fish monger if they sell fresh seagreens, or if they know of a mussel or oyster farmer who grows them. There are a lot of people who are interested in growing seagreens, so the more you ask for them, the more encouragement they'll have to dive in and make a go of it, and that's a good thing.

FROZEN SEAGREENS

With every passing month it becomes easier to find seagreens in your grocer's freezer section. Do not be put off by frozen products, as there is no significant difference in quality between frozen and fresh products (see "Fresh versus Frozen Seagreens," opposite column). The greatest benefit of using frozen seagreens is the reduced risk of spoilage—and you can use the product whenever inspiration strikes. Soon, I hope seagreens will be as easy to buy as spinach and kale. For those of you who can't find it just yet, ask your grocer to stock it.

You can also find frozen kelp online at www.oceanapproved.com/buy-kelp.

Frozen seagreens are quickly blanched in water and then vacuum packed at the peak of quality. The leaves are a vibrant green, mild in flavor, cut into a variety of shapes, and ready to serve right out of the package.

BLANCHING SEAGREENS

Although most fresh-frozen kelp products have been preblanched, you can use a simple method at home to soften the fronds and mellow the flavor before adding seagreens to recipes such as smoothies. To process fresh unblanched kelp, bring a large pot of salted water (seawater is even better) to a boil. Using tongs, gently lower the kelp, one frond at a time, into the pot. Hold it under the water for a few seconds until it turns bright

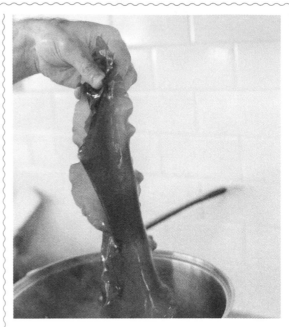

green and then remove it. You can dunk the kelp in cold water to chill it, or add it directly to your recipe.

VOLUME AND PRICE OF SEAGREENS VERSUS FARMED GREENS

Seagreens in dried form can seem skimpy compared to luxurious fluffy salad greens, such as arugula or spinach. However, when seagreens are cooked, the cells do not break down and release water; consequently, the volume of the cooked product stays consistent with fresh greens. So while seagreens may seem significantly more expensive than traditional bagged greens, such as lettuces, the reality is that you end up with equal value by virtue of decreased water loss in the cooking of seagreens. In fact, by volume, cooking seagreens results in a far greater presence in a dish than wilting farmed greens, such as spinach or kale. This is true of rehydrated frozen or fresh seagreens. So don't be put off by the comparatively higher prices, as the value is nearly equal. Given the versatility of seagreens, finding comfortable and even innovative ways to incorporate them into our diet is an exercise in creativity.

FRESH/FROZEN = HOW MUCH REHYDRATED?

Although it is not exact, this guide will help you figure out how to substitute fresh seagreen products with dried ones. Quantities vary. For example, kelp is thick and robust in texture, while dulse is light and feathery. Flavor is also a variable because there is great diversity in the strength and potency of seagreens:

• FOR SOUPS, STEWS, STOCKS: 1 pound fresh = 2 ounces dried

• FOR SALADS: Fresh is really the way to go in terms of providing bulk, although dried seagreens are wonderful when used as a garnish, so these are not necessarily comparable.

• IN SMOOTHIES: 2 ounces (about ¼ cup) fresh = 1 teaspoon dried

• IN BAKED DISHES: The recipes are so precise that I don't recommend much substituting; however, powdered seagreens make a tasty and nutritious substitution for flour. The ratio is generally one part seagreens to two parts flour by volume, given the strength. Use only up to ¼ cup per recipe.

POTENTIAL HAZARDS

Because seagreens are a product of their environment, they are of course influenced by factors in that environment. Just as vegetables can absorb nutrients or toxins from the soil, so too can seagreens absorb nutrients and toxins from the water. It's very important that seagreens are harvested where the water quality is tested and safe for consumption. Given the incredible variety of seagreens that exist in the ocean, it's best to stick to varieties that are well known and commonly used in cooking. I recommend sticking to domestic products and those that come from waters that have been tested. Before incorporating seagreens into your diet, check the resources on page 150 for the most recent and up-to-date information.

HOW TO REHYDRATE SEAGREENS

Given that the most commonly available form of seagreens is dried, an important first step for many preparations is to reinvigorate the character, texture, and flavor of the seagreens. This is especially important if you are using seagreens in a raw preparation, such as a salad or marinated dish. Seagreens can be rehydrated in almost any form of liquid, which serves three purposes:

- (1) to remove any caked salt or other minerals that are deposited on the surface of seagreens during the drying process, giving you greater control over the final seasoning of a dish;

- (2) to flavor seagreens, as they can absorb additional flavors from whatever liquid is used; and

- (3) to make seagreens pliable and appropriately textured for various dishes.

While tepid water is the most common liquid used for this purpose, I like to play around with combinations, such as acidulating the water with lemon juice or vinegar, or adding a touch of white wine or sherry—but don't go overboard with these additions, as the flavor can be intense. The softened seagreens, accented by any added flavors and their own flavor gently smoothed, are now ready for any application you choose.

When making broths with seagreens or adding them to soups, a presoak is unnecessary.

To rehydrate seagreens:

1. Place the desired amount of dried seagreens in a bowl or pot.

2. Warm enough water and/or flavored liquid to cover the dried greens.

3. Pour the liquid over the greens and ensure that they are fully submerged by using a plate or other food-safe item to weigh them down.

4. Let the seagreens soak for at least ten minutes, then check to see if they have fully rehydrated. If more time is needed, replace the weight and check again every five minutes.

5. Once the seagreens are fully soaked, pour off the liquid and let the seagreens drain in a colander. If desired, reserve the soaking liquid, as it can be used for a number of purposes.

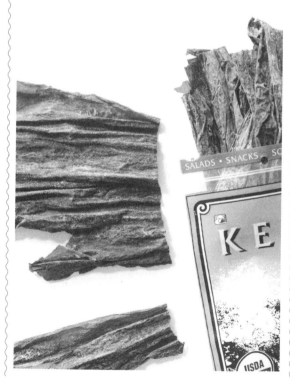

COOKING WITH SEAGREENS

Just as seagreens can be made into a deliciously nuanced broth, they can also be used to create a delicious liquid in which to cook vegetables. This is especially convenient and economical if you are at the shore and have access to clean seagreens, particularly rockweed. (If gathering your own seagreens, make sure you harvest them in accordance with local regulations.) Dried seagreens such as kelp also make for a compelling accent to any cooked vegetable. To cook vegetables, bring a large pot of heavily salted water to a boil and add seagreens. You should rinse fresh seagreens before adding them to the pot in order to remove any grit or tiny shells. Use this liquid to cook corn, potatoes, carrots, sausage, or anything else you'd care to boil. It will imbue these foods with the delicious, magical flavor of the sea.

WHEN SEAGREENS ARE CALLED FOR, WHICH TYPE SHOULD BE USED?

The recipes in this book are designed to be flexible in terms of the type of seagreen or seagreen product that can be used. In most cases any variety of seagreen will work. The exception is when you are making a broth where the deeply concentrated flavor of a dried product is needed and cannot be adequately replaced with fresh product. If you substitute dried-and-rehydrated seagreens for fresh in dishes such as salads, be aware that these products are far more intense in flavor than fresh seagreens, and powdered seagreens are even stronger in flavor.

SMALL PLATES

As seagreens have strong flavors and their nutritional qualities are potent, it is not optimal, from a culinary point of view, to serve them as a full course. With very few exceptions, the flavors of seagreens are most flattering when used in a mélange of flavors, which helps to bring their distinctive qualities into balance. And because most of us are not really used to the flavors of seagreens in our regular dietary repertoire, you're far more likely to enjoy them as a component of your cooking rather than as the centerpiece.

SEAGREENS AND COOKING TIMES

The flavors of seagreens are quite nuanced and, in most species, quite delicate. Cooking seagreens for only a brief time ensures that their subtle bouquet is preserved and doesn't get lost in a dish. Seagreens can become quite bitter if they are cooked too long. It is important to be particularly mindful of this when you are making stocks: the soft flavor of the seagreens will begin to diminish after about half an hour or more of cooking. This first phase of extracting the flavor of seagreens in a broth gives you the clearest, most elegant flavor, with a light, bright, and ebullient personality. After this initial preparation, however, seagreens do not go to waste, as they can be used for salads and other dishes. The stock can be used for multiple recipes, including miso soup, the classic dish served in sushi restaurants the world over. This delicious, warming broth is made by simmering seagreens, straining them, then adding bonito flakes and miso (a paste made from fermented soybeans and barley or rice malt). While this fortified broth has less clarity than the initial preparation, it has a deeper, balanced, meaty flavor that provides an ideal platform for additional ingredients. This broth is a delightful medium for poaching chicken breasts or delicate fillets of fish such as flounder.

SEAGREENS AND SMOKE

Seagreens have varying quantities of iodine, which can make it difficult to pair with smoke, as the combination can result in a slightly tinny flavor. The same is true with the pairing of smoke and ingredients such as crab. However, some seagreens are incredibly elegant when lightly smoked during the drying process; a perfect marriage between woods and water, the rustic, sultry tones of the smoke reminiscent of a driftwood bonfire create a distinctly romantic flavor.

It's possible to apply a very gentle smoke to seagreens that you have rehydrated, especially dulse or kombu, as these take on rustic flavors better than others. The wood that you choose is of the utmost importance, as you need a soft, mild-tempered smoke to flatter and enhance the seagreens. Any orchard wood, such as apple or, my favorite, peach, is the best, in my opinion. Oak, pecan, and alder are all great options. I suggest avoiding bold, sometimes brashly flavored smoke coaxed from hickory or mesquite, as these can potentially bring ruin to the delicate flavors that you are trying to enhance from seagreens.

When smoking rehydrated or even fresh seagreens, just a very brief application of smoke is all that you need. The porous structure of seagreens absorbs the smoke quite readily, and all you are aiming for is to impart just a whisper of smoke. Think of it much like applying perfume. There should be just enough scent so as to be alluring and to captivate the attention of those around you, causing them to wonder exactly who is the source of such a beguiling and attractive scent. It should not be like hopping on the elevator with someone who thinks that it's their duty to impose their perfume on the world. Such is the difference if you're not careful with your application of smoke.

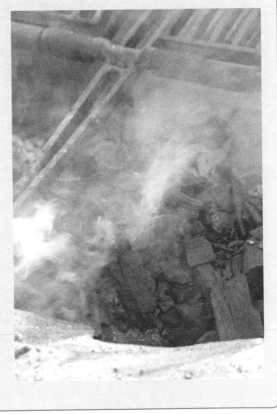

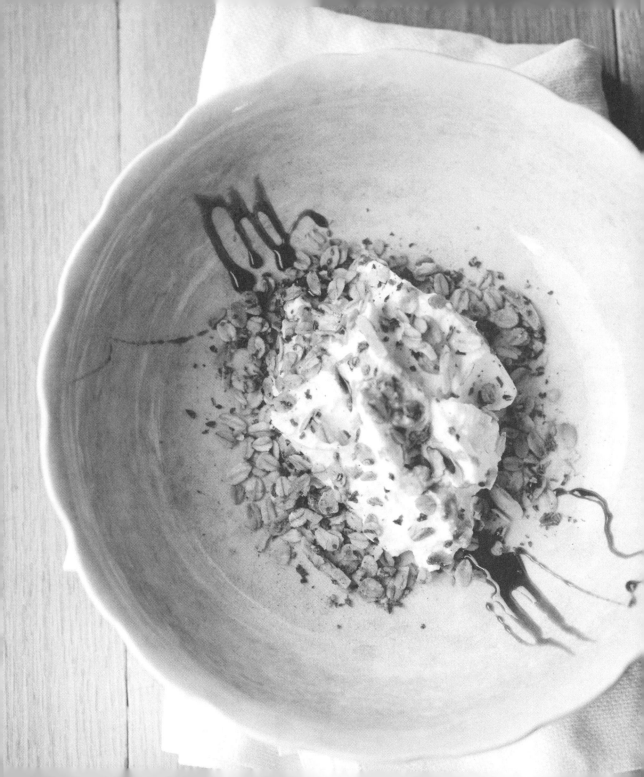

CHAPTER 6

BREAKFAST

What a way to start your day: seagreens for breakfast! Seagreens provide a great dose of dietary fiber, so a nice portion of them in the morning lends staying power to the energy you are looking for from a hearty breakfast. We're all very familiar with the presence of kale or spinach in an omelet, or asparagus in a frittata, so we shouldn't be scared of a little green in our first meal of the day. In all market forms, seagreens can find a place in just about any breakfast meal. Seagreens make a great addition to egg dishes, smoothies, shakes, teas, and even the granola you sprinkle over yogurt—and hey, you can also throw seagreens into your breakfast booze, by following the Bloody Mary recipe on page 63. If you love quiche or burritos for the first meal of the day, you'll find some great recipes here to incorporate seagreens in your favorite breakfast foods.

SEAGREENS SMOOTHIES

Seagreens, in almost all their forms, are far more savory than they are sweet. But through creative pairings and uses, seagreens can blend seamlessly into smoothies, which we commonly understand to be on the sweet side. Any type of seagreen will work in a smoothie—fresh, frozen, dried and rehydrated, flaked, powdered. I've given some recommendations in the recipes that follow to give you an idea of how seagreens can be incorporated into smoothies, but feel free to mix and match. When you add seagreens to smoothies, it's important to know that a small amount goes a long way, especially when you're using dried seagreens, which have an intense, concentrated flavor.

Smoothies aren't just about sweet; they are also all about variety. Choosing diverse fruits and vegetables and combining them in a creative mixture can bring incredible nutritional benefits and convenience to your daily routine. One of the keys to making a successful smoothie is to plan ahead. Just grabbing whatever's available in the fridge, while you are in the midst of the morning rush, is usually not an enjoyable experience, but you can get a jump on the process if you take a few minutes the night before

OPPOSITE: **Spiced Nut and Seagreens Granola, page 64**

to put together the ingredients for the next morning's preparation. I keep a large quantity of bagged, frozen fruit on hand at all times. Each evening, I pull out a handful of whatever fruit currently inspires me and put it in a bowl to defrost overnight. Oatmeal, instant quinoa breakfast flakes, and the like are some of my favorite ingredients that add plenty of fiber to a smoothie. If you add them to the mixture while you're processing it, however, the resulting texture of the smoothie can be grainy and unappealing. To get around this, I add the oatmeal to a bowl of defrosting fruit and liquid the night before. This softening method is similar to the technique used in making muesli, a northern European dish, where oatmeal is soaked overnight, resulting in a hearty cold cereal that is ready to eat the next morning. It's important to choose quick-cooking or instant grain varieties, as slow-cooking products may not fully soften just by soaking. You also want to avoid sweetened, packaged cereals, as these contain lots of artificial flavorings and sugars that have no place in your

FROZEN FRUIT

A large amount of the fruit grown in the United States comes from regions that are often far away from the consumer. In order to withstand the rigors of transportation and the time it takes to get from the plant to the marketplace, the fruit is picked when it is underripe. Consequently, the fruit does not develop its full nutritional profile and flavor. One way to ensure that you are getting the best quality and most nutritious fruit is to shop for it in the frozen food aisle.

Frozen fruit is far less delicate than fresh fruit and can withstand travel far better, resulting in more nutritious product that is often far less expensive, too. Fruit destined for the freezer is picked at the peak of ripeness, when flavors are fully developed, and is frozen within hours of being picked; thus its pristine quality is preserved. An additional benefit to using frozen fruit is convenience: it's available to you straight from your freezer, just when you need it, and allows you to take just what you need for a given preparation and safely keep the rest until you need it. Fresh fruit, on the other hand, must be used within a limited time frame after you buy it. Buying frozen fruit can also save money: you don't throw as much of it away simply because you didn't eat it in time. Because it is less perishable, frozen fruit can give you all the benefits of diversity: with five or more different kinds of fruit that are easily accessible, you can get creative with your smoothies and stave off boredom, one of the main reasons for stopping a perfectly good, healthy habit.

wholesome smoothie. This is a great way to add fiber, which will slow down the absorption of all the nutrients in the drink and give you lasting energy throughout the morning.

The soaking process that applies to oatmeal and quick or instant grains also works well with any dried seagreen that is added to a smoothie. Given time to rehydrate in fruit juices or other liquids, not only does its flavor mellow into the recipe, but its texture also softens and integrates more easily into the final product. Nuts are another great ingredient that you can soak and soften before adding them to a smoothie. The night before, bring a small amount of water to a boil, add the nuts or dried seagreens, and let them sit in the water overnight to hydrate and soften. This will result in a much finer-textured purée in your smoothie.

HOW TO MAKE A GREAT SEAGREEN SMOOTHIE

There's no easier way to start off your day or power through an afternoon than with a seagreen smoothie. To make it supersmooth, blend your greens in liquid first. Then add fruit (frozen fruit works beautifully) and blend again. Add in any extras and pulse to combine all the ingredients.

The Best Seagreens To Use

Frozen seagreens are a little more concentrated than fresh seagreens and have a milder flavor when compared to dried products. Most seagreen flakes have a bit of salinity and can be wonderful when used with nuts to make a more savory protein shake. If you're using a seagreen powder or flakes, such as the Maine Coast Sea Vegetables flaked dulse, start with 1 teaspoon per serving. I've found 2 teaspoons to be the average for each smoothie, but you may need to play around a little with amounts, since different powders vary in potency. You may also discover great fruit combinations that pair particularly well with the distinct marine tang of seagreen powder.

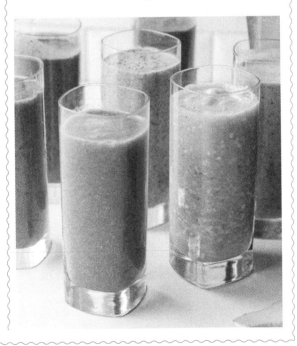

Extras For Seagreen Smoothies

- Nuts or nut butter

- Avocado

- Flaxseeds

- Chia seeds

- Ginger

- Vanilla

- Sweeteners as needed: try dates, honey, maple syrup, agave nectar

BASIC SEAGREEN SMOOTHIE

SERVES 1

1 cup liquid (almond or coconut milk, or yogurt)

½–1 cup fresh or frozen seagreens or 2 teaspoons seagreen powder or flakes

½ banana

1½ cups frozen fruit (blueberries, diced mango, diced pineapple, etc.)

1. Blend the liquid with the seagreens until smooth.

2. Add the remaining ingredients and blend together until smooth.

AVOCADOS

Avocados are the perfect addition to smoothies and salads as they add a rich texture. Their velvety and healthy fats melt into purées and add a luxurious quality to crunchy, peppery greens. They pair particularly well with fruits that have crunch to them, such as apples or pears. Avocados give you plenty of fiber, vitamin K, vitamin E, niacin, vitamin C, and potassium, too. The fats in avocado, though high in calories, are monounsaturated fats, which are heart-healthy. They also have a small amount of heart healthy polyunsaturated omega-3 fatty acids.

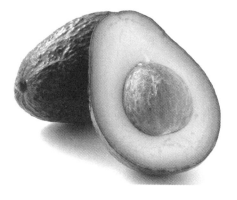

SHAMROCK SHAKE

SERVES 1

- ¾ cup coconut milk
- ¼ cup fresh or frozen seagreens, such as sugar kelp
- ¼ cup fresh mint leaves, picked
- 2 dates, pitted
- ½ banana
- ½ teaspoon vanilla
- 2 ice cubes

1. Blend the liquid with the seagreens and mint until smooth.

2. Add the remaining ingredients and blend together until smooth.

FROZEN SEAGREEN CUBES

To make your own smoothie cubes, blend 1 cup fresh sugar kelp or an equal amount of rehydrated kelp with enough water to liquefy and freeze in ice cube trays. One cube is the right amount for one smoothie.

MIXED FRUIT SUPER GREEN

SERVES 1

- 1 cup coconut milk
- 2 teaspoons kelp powder
- ¼ cup spinach
- ½ cup cherries
- ½ cup blueberries
- ½ banana

1. Blend the liquid with the seagreens and spinach until smooth.

2. Add the remaining ingredients and blend together until smooth.

MANGO MARGARITA

SERVES 1

- 1 cup coconut milk
- 2 teaspoons kelp powder
- 1 cup fresh spinach
- 1 cup frozen mango, diced
- ½ cup frozen pineapple, diced
- ½ teaspoon fresh ginger

1. Blend the liquid with the seagreens and spinach until smooth.

2. Add the remaining ingredients and blend together until smooth.

CHERRY MINT

SERVES 1

- 1   cup milk or yogurt
- 2   teaspoons dulse flakes, rehydrated in ¼ cup warm water
- ¼   cup fresh mint leaves, picked
- 1   cup frozen sweet dark cherries

1. Blend the liquid with the seagreens and mint until smooth.

2. Add the remaining ingredients and blend together until smooth.

NUT BUTTER AND JELLY

SERVES 1

- 1   cup unsweetened almond milk
- 2   teaspoons dulse flakes, rehydrated in ¼ cup water
- 1   cup strawberries
- 1   banana
- 2   tablespoons almond or peanut butter

1. Blend the liquid with the seagreens until smooth.

2. Add the remaining ingredients and blend together until smooth.

MINT

Oh, how I love me some mint. Let's start by talking about the many forms of mint—pineapple mint, orange mint, chocolate mint, peppermint, spearmint, and even catnip are making their way into fine dining. But to me none of these mints are worth more than a curious nod and a little experimentation. Not that these forms of mint are bad in and of themselves, but the traditional mint, the one most commonly found in stores, is such a sublime and beautifully elevating ingredient. To my mind, it is equal to salt and lemon juice in its power to strengthen and make beautiful almost any dish it touches.

My use of mint is quite ubiquitous in recipes, including seagreens, where it is the perfect addition to bring together turf ingredients with flavors of the surf. You'll find that many recipes in this book call for mint as a raw addition to salads and sandwiches, as well as a finishing ingredient to be steeped into soups and broths. And in recipes where mint is not specifically called for, go ahead and give it a try— its beauty is never overwhelming.

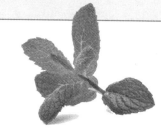

PEACH MELBA

SERVES 1

1 cup water

  Juice of 1 lemon

2 teaspoons kelp powder

½ cup raspberries

1 cup sliced peaches

1. Blend the water and lemon juice with the seagreens until smooth.

2. Add the remaining ingredients and blend together until smooth.

CHOCO-CADO

SERVES 1

1 cup unsweetened almond milk

2 teaspoons kelp powder

1 banana

½ avocado

2 tablespoons cacao powder

2 ice cubes

1. Blend the liquid with the seagreens until smooth.

2. Add the remaining ingredients and blend together until smooth.

PIÑA COLADA

SERVES 1

1 cup coconut milk or water

2 teaspoons kelp powder

1½ cups pineapple

2 tablespoons unsweetened coconut flakes

1. Blend the liquid with the seagreens until smooth.

2. Add the remaining ingredients and blend together until smooth.

PROTEIN PUNCH

SERVES 1

¼ cup rolled oats

1 cup unsweetened almond milk

1 cup fresh or frozen kelp

2 tablespoons almond or peanut butter

6 dates, pitted

1 tablespoon chia seeds

1. Soak the oats in almond milk at least 1 hour or overnight.

2. Blend the oats and milk with the seagreens until smooth.

3. Add the remaining ingredients and blend together until smooth.

OTHER DRINKS

TOMATO-VEGGIE

SERVES 4

This classic mix of vegetables, puréed together into a thick, yet still sippable drink, is made all the more interesting with the addition of seagreens, which lend their characteristic umami flavor to the mix and provide much of the salt. Many store-bought vegetable juices can be very high in sodium, as it requires quite a lot of salt to make tomato juice taste delicious. This is where the element of umami really steps in, pulling out meaty flavors and accentuating the natural sweetness of the ingredients. It brings out so much character that you don't have to add more salt. Sea lettuce in its powdered form is the best seagreen to use for this drink, as it doesn't result in any flecks that can be distracting and, honestly, a little off-putting. Given its soft, mellow personality, sea lettuce is the perfect green for blending.

I add olive oil to this recipe, as the lycopene in tomatoes is made more bioavailable in the presence of this monounsaturated fat. Oh, and it's delicious, too.

2   (14 ounce) cans fire-roasted tomatoes
1   stalk celery
1   cup spinach, firmly packed
4   tablespoons olive oil
1   small beet or ½ cup beet juice
¼   bunch parsley
1   tablespoon Worcestershire sauce
2   tablespoons kelp powder
3   cups water
    Juice of 1 lemon
    Salt
    Hot sauce

1. Combine all of the ingredients except the salt and hot sauce in a Vitamix blender and process on high speed.

2. Taste and adjust the seasoning with hot sauce and salt.

3. Strain for a thinner consistency if desired.

4. Chill and serve over ice.

DIETARY FIBER AND SUGAR ABSORPTION

Beet and carrot juices, while very tasty, are also high in natural sugars. In the juicing process these sugars are separated from the dietary fiber, which in its whole form has the effect of slowing the absorption rate of these sugars.

BLOODY MARY

SERVES 4

Who says nutrition can't come with booze? This version of the vegetable juice cocktail is punctuated with Worcestershire sauce, hot sauce, and the wholly unique bite of horseradish. And hey, I even add in a can of anchovies, as I am particularly partial to their flavor—their nutrition and their salty character adds seasoning to the drink as well. I prefer gin with this Bloody Mary, rather than the traditional vodka, as the juniper flavor so commonly found in gin flatters the seagreen-tomato combination.

1   *recipe Tomato-Veggie (see page 62)*

1   *(2 ounce) can anchovies*

4   *teaspoons horseradish sauce*

    Juice of 1 lemon

4   *tablespoons Worcestershire sauce*

1½ *ounces gin or vodka per serving*

    Hot sauce

    Salt

1. Combine all ingredients in a Vitamix blender and purée until smooth.

2. Taste the seasoning and adjust with hot sauce and salt if needed.

3. Serve over ice.

TEAS AND TISANES

• A great way to gain some of the nutritive value of seagreens is to brew them. Simply steep any type of regular or spicy herbal tea with a leaf or two of dried sea lettuce or a few flakes of dried kelp. Teas and tisanes with fruity components tend to pair exceedingly well with the soft flavors of the seagreens. Rooibos tea makes a particularly nice pairing. Steep the seagreens for the same amount of time as is called for in the tea.

• True teas are made from the leaf of the *Camellia sinensis* plant. While made in a similar fashion and sharing the name *tea*, herbal teas or tisanes are not technically teas at all. Herbal teas such as chamomile, rooibos, and hibiscus teas are made from dried plants, spices, herbs, and even fruits. Traditionally teas and tisanes were consumed for medicinal purposes.

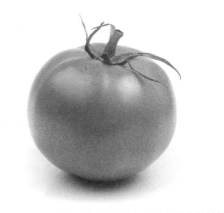

WELLNESS TEA

MAKES ABOUT 9½ CUPS

This is a tea I make for my wife whenever she begins to have even an inkling of illness. It's a wonderful way to soothe a sore throat or simply to use as a restorative tea. I use maple syrup, as it's plentiful in my area, but honey works just as well, or even molasses for those who like a bold flavor.

2   *quarts water*

1   *cup lemon juice*

2   *cinnamon sticks*

½   *cup maple syrup, or more or less to taste*

1   *palm-sized sheet of kombu*

1   *generous pinch cayenne*

1. Bring all ingredients to a simmer and let steep for at least 20 minutes.

2. Strain and serve or keep warm until needed.

DID YOU KNOW?
BLACK TEA AND GREEN TEA

Black tea and green tea are made from the same plant. Black teas are fermented, while green teas are not.

HEARTY BREAKFAST FARE

Seagreens pack a delicious, nutritional punch to start the day. Add them to your breakfast repertoire for an energy boost and to help keep the most important meal of the day as interesting as it can be. The fiber will also help to keep you feeling full for hours to come.

SPICED NUT AND SEAGREENS GRANOLA

MAKES ABOUT 6 CUPS

This breakfast classic can be enjoyed anytime during the day. It is packed full of nutritious ingredients. The addition of seagreens here is barely noticeable beyond its nutritive properties. This granola can be made thicker, into clumps, with the addition of more maple syrup—or molasses or honey, if you don't care for maple syrup. The sweeter, clumpier version of this granola makes a great snack for a hike, but the lower-sugar version is absolutely delicious served over Greek yogurt for an easy breakfast.

4   *cups rolled oats*

½   *cup slivered almonds*

½   *cup chopped walnuts*

½ cup flaxseed meal

4 tablespoons dulse flakes

2 teaspoons ground cinnamon

⅓ cup extra light olive oil or melted coconut oil

⅔ cup pure maple syrup (or molasses or honey)

¼ teaspoon salt

1. Preheat the oven to 350°F. Mix the oats, almonds, walnuts, flaxseed meal, dulse flakes, and cinnamon in a large bowl.

2. Stir the olive or coconut oil, maple syrup, and salt together in a small bowl.

3. Pour the oil mixture over the oat mixture and stir to coat evenly. Spread the resulting mixture evenly onto a parchment-lined baking sheet.

4. Bake until lightly browned, about 40 minutes.

5. Cool completely before breaking into chunks. Store in an airtight container.

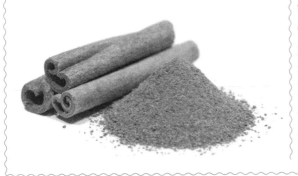

KELP AND FETA OMELET

SERVES 1

We are all familiar with spinach and feta cheese omelets—the flavors of the soft, earthy spinach pair gorgeously with the incredible salty tang of feta in a great classic dish. In this recipe, seagreens are a straight substitute for spinach. The addition of fresh cracked pepper helps to punctuate the flavor of the greens. This dish is particularly delicious with a dollop of fresh tomato salsa on top.

3 eggs, beaten

   Salt

½ tablespoon butter

¼ ounce dried kelp, rehydrated, or ½ cup fresh or frozen seagreens, chopped

1 ounce crumbled feta cheese

1. Season the eggs very lightly with salt.

2. In a 6-inch nonstick sauté pan, heat the butter over medium heat.

3. Add the eggs. Stir for about a minute until the eggs begin to lightly set. Allow the eggs to set and form a smooth surface. Have patience with this as the eggs slowly cook from the bottom up.

4. Add the seagreens and feta, allowing them to warm through as the eggs cook. Fold the omelet and serve immediately.

BREAKFAST BURRITO

SERVES 2

Breakfast burritos are amazingly popular. They are easy to do for a crowd, as many of the components can be made in bulk and assembled when family is gathered. The good thing about a burrito is that you can fill it with nearly any combination of ingredients to create a unique meal.

4 corn tortillas

½ tablespoon butter

3 eggs, beaten

¼ cup black beans, drained and rinsed

¼ cup dulse flakes, rehydrated, or ½ cup fresh or rehydrated kelp

Salt

2 tablespoons sour cream

¼ cup fresh salsa

1. In a dry nonstick pan, heat the corn tortillas two at a time, stacked. Once they are warmed through, keep in a warm location.

2. Add the butter to the pan and scramble the eggs.

3. When the eggs are almost fully cooked, add the black beans and seagreens and finish cooking.

4. Season lightly with salt.

5. Spoon the egg mixture into the warm tortillas, fold in the sides, roll into burrito shapes, and top with a dollop of sour cream and salsa.

ASPARAGUS AND DULSE QUICHE WITH GOAT CHEESE

SERVES 4–6

Quiche is one of the great breakfast treats, especially for entertaining. You can make it the night before, and in the morning the promise of a delicious breakfast will lure you out of bed. The asparagus keeps its bright green color while the dulse adds beautiful flecks of purple.

4 eggs, beaten

1 cup half-and-half

Salt and pepper

2 tablespoons dulse flakes

1 pound asparagus, blanched and chopped

1 (9 inch) unbaked pie crust

4 ounces goat cheese, crumbled

1. Preheat the oven to 350°F. In a medium bowl, whisk together the eggs and half-and-half.

2. Season with salt and pepper.

3. Add the dulse flakes.

4. Place the asparagus in the pie crust. Pour the egg mixture over the asparagus.

5. Bake for 35–40 minutes, until set in the center.

6. Crumble the goat cheese over the top.

7. Allow to stand at least 20 minutes before serving.

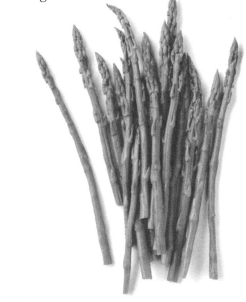

FRITTATA WITH SWEET POTATO AND SEA LETTUCE
SERVES 2

A frittata is basically the lazy man's omelet, which is just fine with me. The colorful ingredients in this recipe are not only jam-packed with great nutrition, they are also beautiful and provide great contrast and textures.

4   eggs, beaten
1   sweet potato, finely diced and boiled until just tender
3   tablespoons cilantro leaves
¼   cup yogurt
1   ounce dried sea lettuce, soaked and chopped
1   tablespoon butter
     Salt

1. Preheat the oven to 350°F. In a medium bowl, mix the eggs, sweet potato, cilantro, yogurt, and sea lettuce.

2. Melt the butter in a small oven-safe pan.

3. Pour the egg mixture into the pan and scramble lightly.

4. Season with salt.

5. Bake in the oven for 12 minutes, or until set.

6. Invert on a plate to serve.

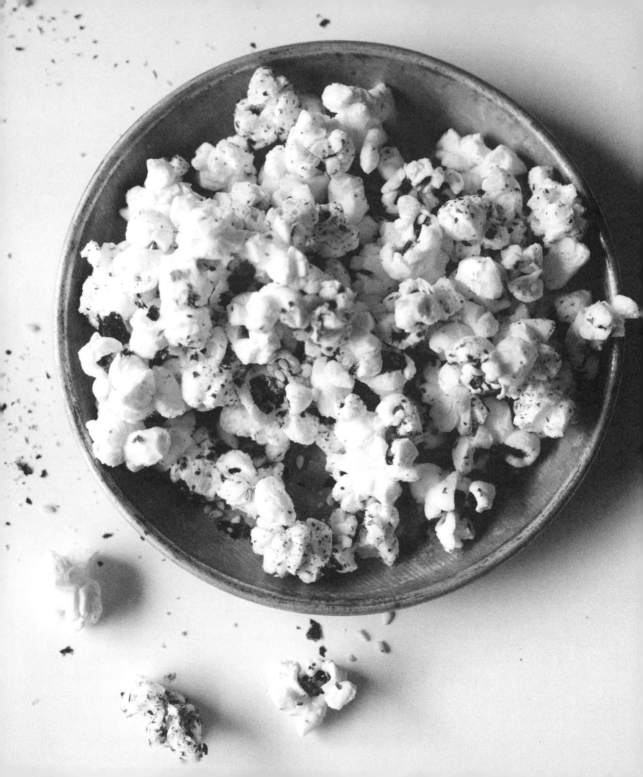

CHAPTER 7

SNACKS

The energy and crunch of the seagreen snacks in this chapter are enough to power you through any afternoon. The seagreen flavor alone is so charismatic and different, it's enough to perk you up. Many of these snacks are elegant and versatile enough to be served at a dinner party, a Super Bowl party, or at home with the family on movie night (try the Furikake Seasoned Popcorn on page 70—delicious!) There's no end to how seagreens can be incorporated into dishes that you already know and love. So dive in.

SMOKY DULSE CHIPS

MAKES ABOUT 40 CHIPS

Just as kale chips have endeared many people to a vegetable that seemed alien at first, dulse chips can be an equally great gateway for anyone who might still be on the fence about seagreens. Making the chips is as simple as a quick sauté in a small amount of oil, or simply baking them without any oil in a moderate oven until they're crisp. You can season the chips with just about anything—some of my favorites are Creole or Old Bay seasoning.

1   tablespoon olive oil, optional
2   ounces regular or applewood-smoked dulse
    Seasoning mix

TO SAUTE:

1. Heat the olive oil over high heat, then add the dulse. Toss to combine.

2. Cook 5–7 minutes over medium heat until crisp.

3. Toss with seasoning mix and let cool before serving.

TO OVEN BAKE:

1. Omit the oil.

2. Spread the dulse on a baking tray.

3. Cook in a 350°F oven for 7–10 minutes, until the dulse begin to crisp.

4. Remove from oven and combine with seasoning mix.

5. Cool before serving.

OPPOSITE: **Furikake Seasoned Popcorn, page 70**

SEAGREEN AND ARTICHOKE DIP

MAKES ABOUT 6 CUPS

This restaurant classic is exceedingly easy to prepare ahead of time, thus perfect for entertaining. It is a dish about which no questions are asked—people just dig in with enthusiasm. In this preparation, most folks would be hard-pressed to note the difference between seagreens and spinach, which makes it a good recipe for introducing seagreens to people who are unfamiliar with them.

- 2 *(8 ounce) packages cream cheese, softened*
- ½ *cup mayonnaise*
- ½ *cup freshly grated Parmesan cheese*
- 2 *(14 ounce) cans marinated artichoke heart quarters, drained and chopped*
- 2 *chipotle chiles in adobo, chopped*
- 1 *ounce nori, rehydrated, drained, and chopped (about 1 cup)*
- ½ *cup heavy cream*
- ½ *cup panko bread crumbs*

1. Preheat the oven to 350°F.

2. Mix together the cream cheese and mayonnaise in a bowl until smooth.

3. Stir in the Parmesan cheese, artichokes, chiles, and nori.

DAIRY PRODUCTS AND SEAGREENS

The old adage that cheese does not pair well with seafood is worth revisiting. To my mind, dairy products and seagreens are often a wonderful pairing. I've found in these recipes that the acidic personality of goat cheese matches beautifully with seagreens, especially rehydrated kombu and dulse. And cream cheese and sour cream provide excellent platforms for the aromatic seagreens in almost any type of casserole. Seagreens substitute well in my take on classic creamed spinach (see page 95).

---

4. Spoon the mixture into a baking dish. Cover with heavy cream, and then sprinkle panko on top.

5. Bake until brown, about 30 minutes.

FURIKAKE SEASONED POPCORN

MAKES ABOUT ¾ CUP FURIKAKE, FOR AS MUCH POPCORN AS YOU CARE TO EAT

Furikake is a wonderful blend of salty, spicy, and savory flavors that, when simmered in a little bit of butter and then drizzled over hot, fresh-popped corn, becomes not only a colorful, unique snack but also a fun way to welcome guests and start conversations at a dinner party.

½ cup raw or toasted sesame seeds

3 sheets nori, dry toasted

3 heaping tablespoons bonito flakes

Coarse popcorn salt

Unpopped popcorn kernels

Melted butter

1. Place ¼ cup sesame seeds in a large bowl.

2. To make the furikake, in a spice grinder, pulse the remaining ¼ cup sesame seeds until powdered. Do not overprocess—you do not want to create a paste.

3. Add the powdered sesame seeds to the whole sesame seeds.

4. Add half the nori to the grinder and pulse until it is a fine powder, and reserve. Pulse the remaining nori into small flakes, and reserve. Pulse the bonito flakes into small flakes. Combine all and season with popcorn salt to taste.

5. Pop the popcorn according to the package directions. Drizzle with butter and dust with furikake.

KATHY'S MULTIGRAIN CRACKERS

MAKES ABOUT 4 DOZEN CRACKERS

This recipe is inspired by the perfect creation of our friend Kathy Heye. To her recipe I've added the smoky touch of dulse. These wisp-thin, crispy crackers are a delight on their own or with just a little bit of goat cheese on top.

3 cups rolled oats

¼ ounce applewood-smoked dulse, finely chopped

2 cups unbleached all-purpose flour

1 cup wheat germ

¾ cup canola oil

⅓ cup brown sugar

1 teaspoon kosher salt, plus more for sprinkling

1½ cups water

1. Preheat the oven to 350°F.

2. In a bowl, combine all ingredients. Mix together until you have a pliable dough.

3. Roll out the dough and place it on two ungreased rimmed cookie sheets.

4. Cut the dough into cracker-sized rectangles. Bake for 30 minutes or until the crackers begin to brown at the edges.

(continued)

5. As the individual crackers brown, take them out of the oven and cool them on a rack.

6. As you remove the fully baked crackers from around the edges of the pan, spread the remaining crackers around the pan so they brown and crisp evenly.

7. Cool before serving.

SEAGREEN GUACAMOLE
SERVES 4

Guacamole, the luxurious purée of buttery avocado brightened by the acidity of lime and aromatic cilantro, is the perfect vehicle for seagreens. Their unique flavor melds beautifully with the other ingredients, adding both nuance and nutrition to this familiar favorite.

Juice of 1 lime
Salt
1   *hot pepper, such as serrano or Fresno, finely diced*
4   *tablespoons powdered sea lettuce or dulse*
1   *bunch cilantro, chopped*
3   *ripe avocados*

1. In a bowl combine the lime juice with the salt, hot pepper, seagreens, and cilantro.

2. Stir to incorporate and let sit for 5 minutes to allow flavors to develop.

3. Slice the avocados in half from top to bottom and rotate one half away from the other to separate them. Sink the heel of the knife into the avocado pit and bang the pit off the knife, using the side of a trash can. This method ensures your safety, as you aren't trying to grip the slippery pit with your hand.

4. While the flesh is still in the peel, cut each half of the avocado into cross sections. This will make the mashing much easier and help keep your guacamole green longer, since you won't be exposing the flesh to much oxygen (which is what gives it a brown color).

5. Using a large spoon, scoop the avocado into the bowl with the other ingredients and mash to combine.

6. Check the seasoning and adjust as needed.

7. Serve with pita chips, tortilla chips, or seagreen crackers (see page 71).

DID YOU KNOW?
BLACK PEPPER

Before spices were available universally, black pepper was so rare and valuable that it was used as currency. Imagine what it must have been like never to have tasted the gentle bite of pepper. It's not a stretch to say that this charismatic and now ubiquitous ingredient was once worth its weight in gold.

DULSE-SPECKLED GOAT CHEESE

SERVES 6

This recipe was inspired by my love of goat cheese, which absorbs the flavors of anything it is paired with and is especially well suited to fresh herbs. Another idea is to roll goat cheese in furikake as an elegant way to add something unique to a traditional cheese platter.

6   ounces goat cheese, softened to room temperature
1   tablespoon dulse flakes or sea lettuce
    Pinch salt
    Cracked pepper
    Juice of ½ lemon
2   tablespoons olive oil

1. Whisk together all ingredients with a fork until well combined.

2. Place in a serving bowl and let it sit for at least 20 minutes before serving.

3. Drizzle with additional lemon juice or olive oil for added elegance.

SEAGREEN ENERGY BARS

MAKES 8 BARS

In our modern world, convenience is king. These energy bars can be made in large batches and will keep up to a week. They provide a huge dose of nutrition-packed energy. Try adding ginger or change up the nuts and dried fruit for variety.

4   tablespoons sea lettuce flakes
¼   cup water
½   cup cashews
8   ounces dried dates, pitted
¼   cup flaxseed meal
2   cups quinoa flakes
2   tablespoons sesame seeds
2   tablespoons dried chopped orange peel
    Pinch salt

1. Preheat the oven to 300°F. Dissolve the sea lettuce flakes in the water.

2. In a Vitamix or other high-powered blender, combine the softened sea lettuce, along with any remaining water, with the cashews and dates until smooth.

3. Mix in all remaining ingredients.

4. Press the mixture into a baking sheet lined with parchment paper.

5. Bake for 2 hours or until dried. Cut into bars and keep in an airtight container.

FLATBREADS

Flatbreads are immensely popular and are easy to make using ready-to-bake pizza doughs available at many grocery stores. There are two main methods for creating the flatbread crust: stovetop and oven.

STOVETOP FLATBREAD

This is the quickest method for making flatbread.

1. Shape the dough into a thin round and place it directly in a nonstick or cast-iron pan over medium-high heat.

2. Press down any air bubbles as they form.

3. Flip the bread once, cooking each side until it has browned nicely, 2–3 minutes per side. Then top as desired.

OVEN-BAKED FLATBREAD

I like to bake flatbreads in an oval-shaped fish pan—the dough that overflows the pan makes for a rustic look. This works best with toppings that require a little bit of baking. I like to use roasted butternut squash and top it off with shaved pecorino cheese and applewood-smoked dulse.

1. Preheat the oven to 400°F. Roll out the dough like a thin pizza. Be sure that any toppings you add cover the surface of the bread, all the way to the edges, to keep the crust from puffing up.

2. Bake the flatbread until the crust is brown, about 10 minutes. Using a dry pan delivers a wonderfully crisp crust.

FLATBREAD WITH BUTTERNUT SQUASH AND SMOKED DULSE

SERVES 6–8

 1 *cup butternut squash, peeled and diced into ½ inch cubes*

 2 *tablespoons extra virgin olive oil*
    Salt

 ½ *ounce smoked dulse*

 1 *ounce pecorino or parmesan*

1. Saute butternut squash in 1 tablespoon olive oil until soft and just brown, cool slightly.

2. Roll out dough and brush with remaining olive oil and season with salt.

3. Top dough with squash and half the dulse.

4. Bake or cook on stovetop until cooked through.

5. Remove from heat and top with remaining dulse and cheese. Serve immediately.

CARAMELIZED ONIONS WITH KOMBU

SERVES 6–8

Caramelizing onions is work, but it is well worth the time. Caramelized onions pair well with goat cheese or feta cheese, and maybe a little toasted quinoa for added crunch—or even anchovies.

Make the flatbread dough, following either preparation as described opposite.

2 cups sliced onion (about 1 large)

½ ounce dried kombu, crumbled

3 tablespoons butter

1½ cups water

1. Make dough according to either method on page 74.

2. Cook the onions and kombu in butter over high heat until they begin to char and turn dark brown.

3. Add 6 tablespoons of the water and reduce heat to medium. Allow onions to cook until they are dry and begin to color again.

4. Repeat three times with 6 more tablespoons of the water at a time until the onions are a rich caramel color and the kombu has been fully hydrated.

GRILLED GARLIC NORI BREAD

SERVES 6–8

Who doesn't love garlic bread? In this recipe, the combination of parsley, Parmesan cheese, and nori is a fun (and delicious) take on the classic preparation.

½ baguette

4 tablespoons extra virgin olive oil

2 tablespoons crumbled nori (or dulse)

2 tablespoons chopped fresh flat-leaf parsley (from about 10 sprigs)

4 cloves garlic, grated on a Microplane™ grater or very finely minced

2 tablespoons grated Parmesan cheese

1. Slice the baguette horizontally, as if for a sandwich, and lay the halves crust-side down on a baking sheet.

2. Mix the olive oil, nori, parsley, garlic, and Parmesan, and whisk to combine. Spread the mixture evenly over the bread. Let it sit for at least 10 minutes for the oil to soak in.

3. Place the bread herb-side up under the broiler set to medium. Cook until the bread begins to brown and the olive oil is sizzling, about 10 minutes. Remove from the broiler and serve immediately.

SUSHI

Now, I'm no sushi master. Indeed, I'm very far from it. Most likely you are in the same boat: a sushi lover, as I am, and a little trepidatious about making the stuff yourself, but willing to give it a shot anyway.

Simply put, sushi is made with vinegar-spiked rice that can be wrapped around or topped by any number of ingredients (traditionally a slice of fish or vegetable) and then wrapped in seaweed. The rice used to make sushi is a short, fat Japanese variety that can be found in many stores. Follow the instructions on the package to prepare it. The grains are prized for their sticky and starchy flavor. The rice, spiked with rice wine vinegar, is truly what makes sushi an art form, and disciples of the great sushi masters spend years learning to make it properly. Will you make it perfectly? I know I don't. Will you make it satisfying and delicious? Probably.

Why is sushi in this book? Because it is wrapped in sheets of the seagreen nori, which is harvested, washed, turned into a paste, and then pressed and rolled into paper-thin sheets. Nori is delicious on its own, toasted with a bit of salt or flavored with teriyaki sauce. Each sheet of nori has a shiny side and a dull, matte side.

For the preparation of sushi, nori sheets are toasted to heighten their flavor. The sheets are then spread with rice on the shiny side (important for preserving the texture and snappy bite of the roll), other ingredients are added, and then all the components are rolled into a tight tubelike form. It is then sliced across the roll to reveal the gorgeous construction of the dark nori sheet, the snow-white rice, and any colorful ingredients that were rolled into the center.

Usually, sushi includes raw fish or vegetables. Before using raw fish, you should familiarize yourself with a great fishmonger or look in the freezer aisle of your local supermarket for high-quality fillets.

I like to add carrot sticks or sweet potato batons that have been softened by boiling them in water and vinegar. Basically, you can add whatever you want to your sushi rolls—whatever looks great at the store.

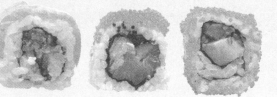

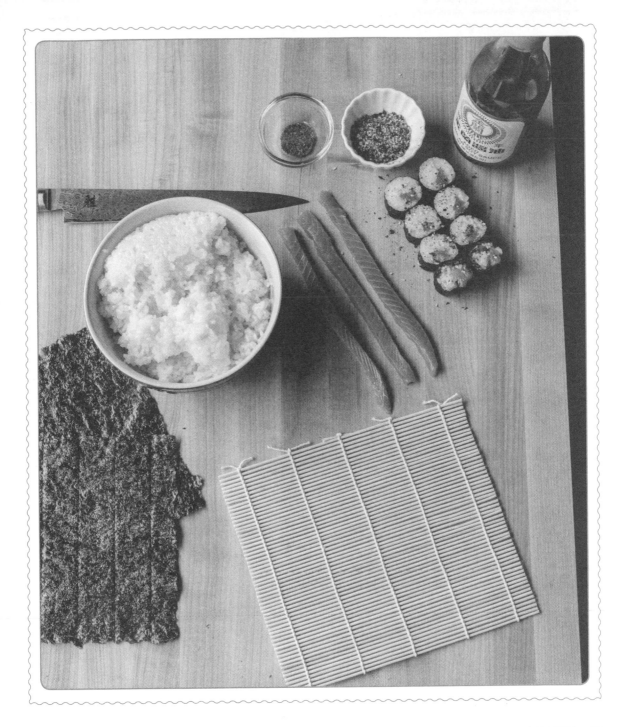

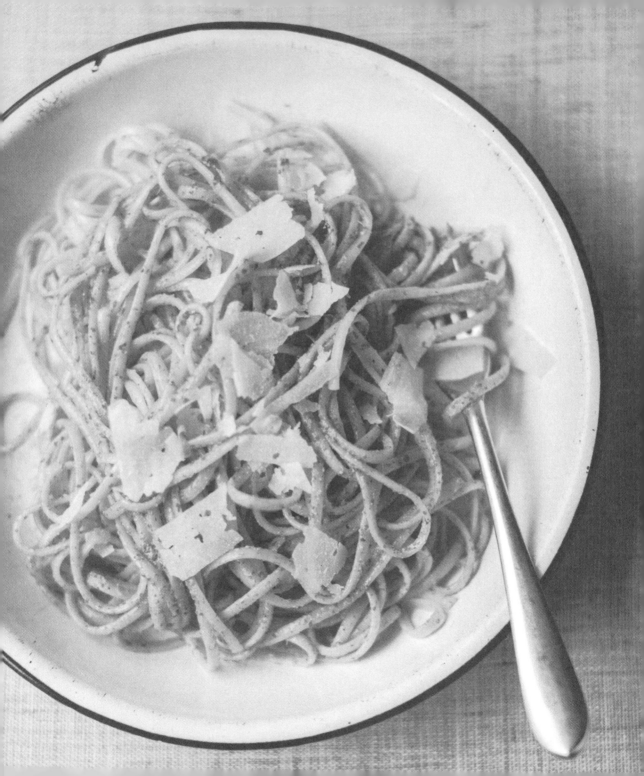

CHAPTER 8

SAUCES, SPICES, AND SIDES

In this chapter, seagreens really come alive, as their umami flavor is front and center in ways that flatter other ingredients. Particularly in sauces, seagreens lend a heavy dose of umami, deepening, strengthening, and enriching the flavors of anything they touch. In side dishes, the greens do much the same, lending a hand to recipes such as Creamed Seagreens (see page 95) or Braised Red Cabbage with Seagreens (see page 97). They are equally delicious stewed, collard style, or sautéed with bacon and apples and onions. Trying any of the recipes in this chapter is a fun way to experiment with and enjoy the wonderful personality of seagreens.

PESTOS

Pestos are wonderfully easy to make. The combination of nuts and herbs that can be used in these fabulous mixtures is near infinite, depending on what you have in your pantry, and they can be used to top off or toss with just about anything, from grilled seafood to cooked pastas, especially soba, Asian buckwheat noodles. Adding pesto to a dish after it is finished cooking allows the residual heat to warm the pesto and bloom its flavors.

KELP, WALNUT, AND GINGER PESTO

MAKES ABOUT 1½ CUPS

1   *cup fresh or frozen kelp, or ½ ounce dried kelp, rehydrated and water reserved*

1½ *teaspoons minced fresh ginger*

1   *small garlic clove*

½   *cup water, plus more as needed for texture*

½   *cup walnuts*

½   *cup extra virgin olive oil*

    Salt

1. Add the kelp, ginger, garlic, and ½ cup water (or ½ cup water from soaking kelp) to a Vitamix blender.

(continued)

2. Purée, adding a little more water as needed.

3. Add the walnuts and extra virgin olive oil. Purée until smooth.

4. Season with salt.

KELP AND CASHEW PESTO
MAKES ABOUT 2 CUPS

1   *clove garlic*

½   *cup water*

1   *cup fresh or frozen kelp, or ½ ounce dried kelp, rehydrated and water reserved*

1   *cup fresh parsley*

½   *cup extra virgin olive oil*

½   *cup cashews*
    Salt

1. Add the garlic and water (use the water from rehydrating the kelp, if you used dried) to a Vitamix blender and purée.

2. Add the kelp and parsley and blend.

3. With the machine running, pour in the olive oil.

4. Add the cashews and continue to purée until smooth.

5. Season with salt.

ROASTED SQUASH HUMMUS WITH CRUNCHY WAKAME
MAKES ABOUT 6 CUPS

This surprisingly delightful dish delivers the same creamy texture that we love so much in traditional chickpea hummus. The combination of sesame (in the form of tahini, a sesame paste available in most grocery stores) and the seagreens is a perfect pairing. If you want, you can add about ¼ cup finely chopped dulse (applewood-smoked dulse would be fabulous); it will leave the hummus slightly less creamy but beautifully flecked with brown-purple bits. In this recipe, I suggest using crumbled dried wakame, as its heady crunch is a perfect counterpoint to the creamy hummus. Any type of thick-skinned winter squash will do in this recipe. My favorites are kabocha, butternut, hubbard, and regular old pumpkin. Serve the hummus with baguette slices. It is equally nice on toasted pita bread or vegetable sticks. The recipe makes enough to serve twice.

1   *winter squash (1–2 pounds)*

½   *cup tahini*
    Juice of 1 lemon

1   *clove garlic, grated on a Microplane grater or very finely minced (optional)*
    Kosher salt

2   *cups extra virgin olive oil*

Freshly grated nutmeg

Chile flakes (optional)

½ *cup crumbled dried wakame*

1 *small baguette, sliced on the bias ½-inch thick; pita bread; or vegetable sticks*

1. Preheat the oven to 325°F. Cut the squash in half lengthwise and remove the seeds. Place it cut-side down in a baking dish with a small amount of water.

2. Cover with aluminum foil and bake for approximately 45 minutes to 1 hour, until the squash is soft to the touch.

3. Remove it from the oven and allow it to cool until you can easily handle it. Using a spoon, scrape the flesh from the skin. Discard the skin.

4. In a food processor, combine the squash, tahini, lemon juice, garlic, and a pinch of salt. Process until mostly smooth.

5. With the processor running, slowly drizzle in the olive oil until you have a finely textured paste.

6. Scrape into a large bowl and garnish with nutmeg, chile flakes, if desired, and the crumbled wakame. Any remaining hummus will keep in the fridge for up to 5 days.

MARINADES AND SAUCES

SEAGREEN AND HERB MARINADE

MAKES ABOUT 1½ CUPS

Use this marinade for any type of seafood, steaks, pork, chicken, or tofu. It's best used with items destined for the grill. Let the food marinate for at least 20 minutes prior to cooking.

½ *bunch parsley, chopped*

½ *bunch mint, chopped*

Juice of 1 lemon

1 *clove garlic, mashed or grated with a Microplane grater*

2 *teaspoons dulse flakes*

1 *cup olive oil*

Salt

1. Combine all ingredients in a food processor and purée until mostly smooth.

(SEA)GREEN GODDESS DRESSING

MAKES ABOUT 1¼ CUPS

Green goddess is a classic American dressing. Its delicious herbal characteristics pair well with everything from chilled seafood and chicken to hearty lettuces such as iceberg and romaine.

1   cup mayonnaise or Greek yogurt

1   (2 ounce) tin oil-packed anchovies

1   bunch tarragon, leaves only

1   bunch parsley, leaves only

    Juice of 1 lemon

    Salt

½   ounce dried kombu, rehydrated in warm water with a dash of lemon juice, then drained

1. Combine all ingredients in a food processor and purée until smooth and bright green. The mixture will be slightly chunky with herbs.

2. Allow it to rest at least 1 hour and up to overnight to allow the flavors to meld.

ANCHOVIES

One of my very favorite ingredients in just about everything is the much-maligned anchovy, which many people were turned off of in their youth thanks to bad pizza featuring the tiny, briny fish. This is unfortunate because a little 2-ounce can of anchovies can add a lot of flavor and a huge punch of omega-3 fatty acids and protein to a dish. Anchovies, like seagreens, need not be a centerpiece and in fact are overwhelming when used as such. Just a few of the fillets melted into butter at the beginning of a dish, or simmered into a soup until they disintegrate, adds all their nutritional benefit, along with enriching flavors, and provide a wonderful and unexpected elegance to a dish. When used together in, say, a seagreen salad with anchovy vinaigrette, the results are stunning.

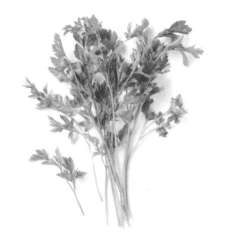

BUTTERMILK, KELP, AND MINT DRESSING

MAKES ABOUT ¾ CUP

This is a favorite recipe from one of my earlier cookbooks, which I've adapted to include seagreens. In this version, powdered kelp or sea lettuce add a richness that draws out the creaminess of the buttermilk and lets the aromatic mint soar. This dressing is perfect for crunchy greens such as romaine and, my favorite, radicchio.

½ tablespoon powdered kelp or 1 tablespoon flaked sea lettuce

1 tablespoon extra virgin olive oil

1 teaspoon Dijon mustard

1 teaspoon sugar

½ cup low-fat buttermilk

Juice of ½ lemon

Leaves from 8 sprigs fresh mint, chopped

Salt

1. Combine the seagreens, olive oil, mustard, sugar, buttermilk, lemon juice, and mint in a bowl and mix together. Allow to sit at room temperature for at least 20 minutes and up to 2 hours so that the flavors combine.

2. Taste for seasoning and adjust with salt if necessary.

TOASTED NORI VINAIGRETTE

MAKES ABOUT ¼ CUP

This vinaigrette is perfect for spicy greens such as arugula or baby mustard greens.

1 clove garlic, grated

1 teaspoon dry mustard powder

1 tablespoon wine vinegar

1 sprig thyme, leaves only

2 teaspoons dried nori flakes

3 tablespoons extra virgin olive oil

Salt

1. Combine all ingredients and whisk to incorporate. Let sit 10 minutes before using.

SEAGREENS AND BREAST HEALTH

Many scientists hypothesize that the low incidence of breast disease in Japanese women can be attributed to frequent consumption of seagreens.

SMOKY DULSE GREMOLATA

MAKES ABOUT ¼ CUP

Gremolata is a wonderfully acidic and pleasant condiment backed with a little bit of bite from garlic. Traditionally used to garnish long-braised dishes such as osso buco, the slightly spicy yet fresh flavors of gremolata become vibrant and heady as they bloom from the heat of a simple grilled chicken breast, steak, roasted fish, or seared tofu.

½ bunch flat-leaf parsley
1 tablespoon finely chopped dried dulse, regular or applewood smoked
  Zest of 1 lemon
1 small clove garlic, grated
  Salt
  Dash ground mace
2 tablespoons extra virgin olive oil, plus more for garnish

1. Chop the parsley until almost fully minced.

2. Add the dulse, lemon zest, and garlic, then finish chopping.

3. Add a touch of salt and the mace. Transfer to a bowl and mix with the olive oil. Let sit for at least 20 minutes before using.

4. Depending on use, add more olive oil if needed.

TANGY SPICED GRAVY

SERVES 8–10

For anyone seeking an alternative to traditional rich turkey or chicken gravy, this lightly thickened version with reduced seagreen stock and flavored with herbs provides a familiar and yet unexpected touch to a holiday meal.

3 cups Vegetable and Seagreen Broth (see page 113)
  Dash amontillado sherry
4 allspice berries
10 black peppercorns
2 sprigs thyme
1 bay leaf
  Slice of fresh ginger
1 teaspoon dulse flakes (smoked is preferable)
  Salt
2 teaspoons cornstarch
2 tablespoons cold water

1. In a large saucepan, combine the broth, sherry, allspice, peppercorns, thyme, bay leaf, ginger, and dulse.

2. Bring to a simmer and reduce by half. Season with salt.

3. Combine the cornstarch with the cold water. Stir to make a paste. Bring the gravy to a full boil and, while whisking, add the cornstarch mixture. Cook at a full boil until the gravy has thickened.

4. Remove from the heat. Strain out the solids and serve.

(SEA)GREEN CURRY SAUCE

MAKES ABOUT 4 CUPS

The herbs in this fresh curry sauce make it light and bright in contrast to the deeply spiced, brooding, and complex flavor of some powder-based dishes. I like to finish it off with lime juice and yogurt, not only to temper some of the heat but also to further accentuate the flavors with a burst of acidity. This green curry sauce can be poured over a simple brown rice pilaf or it can be used as a delicious base liquid in which to braise seafood, tofu, or chicken.

4   *tablespoons butter*
1   *tablespoon ground cumin*
1   *tablespoon ground coriander*
1   *onion, grated*
1   *bulb fennel, grated*
1   *half-inch knob fresh ginger, grated*
2   *garlic cloves, grated*
1   *stalk lemongrass*
1   *bay leaf*
1   *star anise pod*
1   *hot pepper, such as jalapeño, sliced in rings*
1   *cup cashews*
3   *cups Chicken and Seagreen Stock (see page 113)*
1   *bunch cilantro*
1   *bunch parsley*
1   *cup fresh or frozen blanched seagreens, or 1 ounce dried, rehydrated seagreens*
    Juice of 1 lime
½   *cup yogurt*
    Salt

1. In a large saucepan, heat the butter with the cumin, coriander, onion, fennel, ginger, garlic, lemongrass, bay leaf, anise, hot pepper, and cashews. Lightly sauté for 15 minutes until the aromas begin to soften.

2. Add the seagreen stock, bring to a boil, and boil for 5 minutes.

3. Remove the lemongrass, bay leaf, and star anise, and discard.

4. Transfer the broth and remaining solids to a Vitamix blender and purée.

5. Add the herbs and seagreens and purée until smooth.

6. Add the lime juice and yogurt, and season with salt.

UMAMI-SPICY MARINARA SAUCE

MAKES ABOUT 1 QUART

This fresh take on the classic sauce combines flavors of sweet and spice. Marinara is a natural vehicle for umami-rich dulse, which enlivens the tomatoes with smoke. This sauce is haunting when paired with whole wheat or quinoa pasta for an easy and nutritious dinner.

- 1 clove garlic, sliced
- 6 tablespoons extra virgin olive oil
- 4 whole Calabrian chiles or chile de árbol (or 2 teaspoons chile flakes)
- 2 tablespoons applewood-smoked (or regular) dulse flakes
- 1 (28 ounce) can diced fire-roasted tomatoes
  Salt

1. Brown the garlic in 4 tablespoons of the olive oil.

2. Add the chiles and dulse flakes and toss to coat in oil.

3. Add the tomatoes and bring to a simmer. Cook down for about 10 minutes. Fish out the peppers or not—depending on who you're having to dinner.

4. Add the remaining 2 tablespoons olive oil, season with salt, and mash the tomato chunks with the back of a wooden spoon.

SEAGREEN BUTTER SAUCE

MAKES ABOUT ¼ CUP

In the world of fine French cuisine, seagreen butter has long been a secret weapon. This sauce is especially delicious when made with a very high-quality European butter, preferably cultured butter with a rich, Parmesan-like scent. Once mixed, let the butter rest long enough for the flavors to meld. Traditionally, it is used to top baked or seared meat or fish after cooking. The heat melts the butter over the food, giving it both visual and aromatic appeal.

- 1 tablespoon flaked dried seagreens, such as dulse
- 1 teaspoon Pernod, or other anise-scented liqueur
- ¼ cup butter, softened
- ½ teaspoon ground allspice
  Salt
  Freshly ground pepper

1. Combine all the ingredients and whip to incorporate.

2. Roll in plastic wrap and refrigerate or freeze until needed.

SEAGREEN SEASONING SALTS

These spicy seagreen/salt combinations are a wonderful way to get some of the nutritive benefits of seagreens into any meal, as they complement just about everything, from a simple chicken breast to baked fish and even roasted or sautéed vegetables.

TO PREPARE: Simply combine all ingredients. Store in an airtight container until ready to use.

CREOLE GRILL SEASONING
MAKES APPROXIMATELY ¼ CUP

- 1 tablespoon dried oregano
- 1 tablespoon smoked sweet paprika
- 1 teaspoon powdered thyme
- 2 teaspoons onion powder
- 1 tablespoon kelp powder
- 1 tablespoon salt

SICILIAN HERB RUB
MAKES APPROXIMATELY ¼ CUP

- 1 tablespoon dried oregano
- 1 teaspoon garlic powder
- ½ teaspoon mace powder
- ½ teaspoon powdered thyme
- 1 teaspoon chile flakes
- 1 tablespoon salt
- 1 tablespoon kelp powder

SPICY FISH RUB
MAKES APPROXIMATELY ¼ CUP

- 1 teaspoon ground cinnamon
- 1 teaspoon ground ginger
- 1 teaspoon onion powder
- 1 teaspoon ground nutmeg
- 1 teaspoon dried oregano
- 1 teaspoon ground chile
- 1 teaspoon powdered thyme
- 2 teaspoons kelp powder
- 2 teaspoons salt

HERBES DE PROVENCE
MAKES APPROXIMATELY ¼ CUP

- 1 teaspoon dried oregano
- ½ teaspoon powdered thyme
- 1 tablespoon salt
- 1 teaspoon ground rosemary
- 1 tablespoon fennel seed
- ¼ teaspoon ground ginger
- 1 teaspoon onion powder
- 2 tablespoons kelp powder

SEXY SALTS

Though seagreens can be high in salt, given that they come from seawater, most recipes in this book call for the addition of salt to help season and flavor the other ingredients because the salt contained in seagreens is often not quite enough. Different culinary salts range from the ubiquitous table salt, which contains iodine for thyroid heath, to the salts more commonly used in professional kitchens such as sea salt and kosher salt. There is also a market for super sexy Maldon flake salts, Hawaiian pink salts, lava born black salt, and, of course, smoked and flavored salts. In my opinion, salt is salt. And the purpose of using salt is to make things taste more like they do. Salt is a flavor enhancer, rather than a flavor addition. Therefore the type of salt is not as important as how you use it. The process of salting is a physical memory. We visually gauge the volume and density of a dish and then pick up a pinch of salt to season. It is this memory of knowing how much seasoning your pinch delivers that is valuable to the cook. So choose your salt, any salt, but choose one. Get to know it. Become very familiar with its properties and use. By perfecting the art of salting with a single salt, you will gain far more than you will sacrifice by the exclusion of other salt options.

- KOSHER SALT is large in volume and has a crunchy flake. It dissolves easily. This is the preferred salt of professional kitchens. It is great for all applications because it adheres well to items like steaks and dissolves well into soups or broths. It also cures foods well as its volume-to-salt ratio is large, thus you can cover a large surface area with a lower amount of salt.

- IODIZED SALT is what you find in salt shakers everywhere. It can be hard to use as its dense crystal dissolves slowly and is potently salty. Using this to appropriately season an item with a large surface area, such as a tomato slice or steak, can be difficult because just a few grains per square inch are enough salt, but it's tough to sprinkle evenly to season properly. That said, this is the salt most people are comfortable with and have become accustomed to using. So if you know how to use it, then by all means do.

- SEA SALT comes in many forms, including sel gris or fleur de sel. While most of the salt we used is mined from deposits in the earth, the largest source of salt covers the largest area of this planet, the oceans. Salt has been made from seawater by the process of evaporation (solar, wind, boiling) ever since humans showed up on the coast. The various mineral components of water from different regions, the different microalgae and microscopic life, and the temperature of the water all give salts

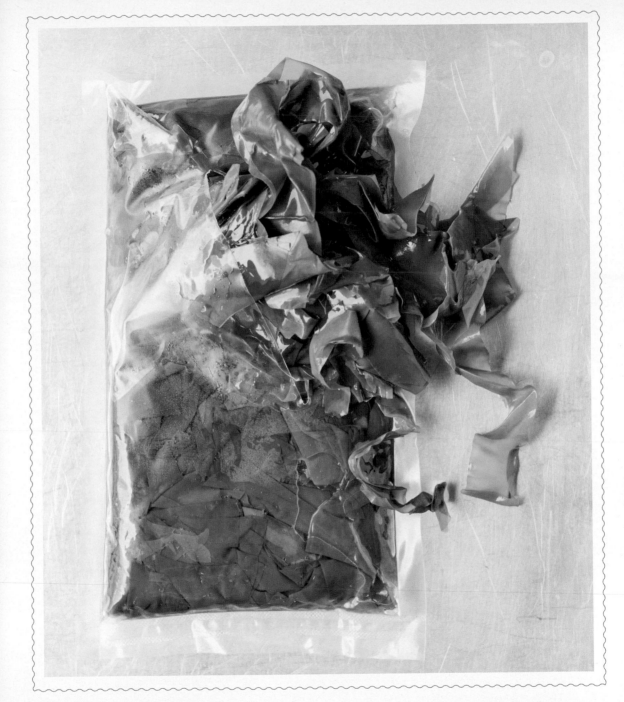

Packaged Frozen Seagreens

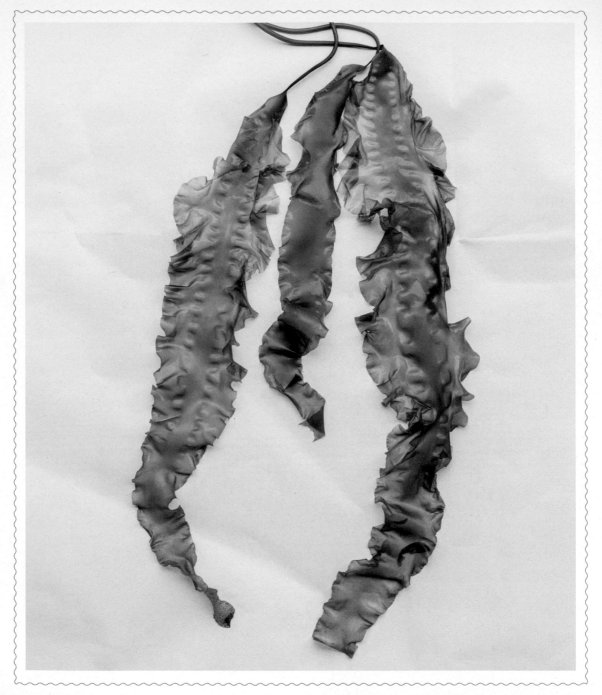

Sugar Kelp

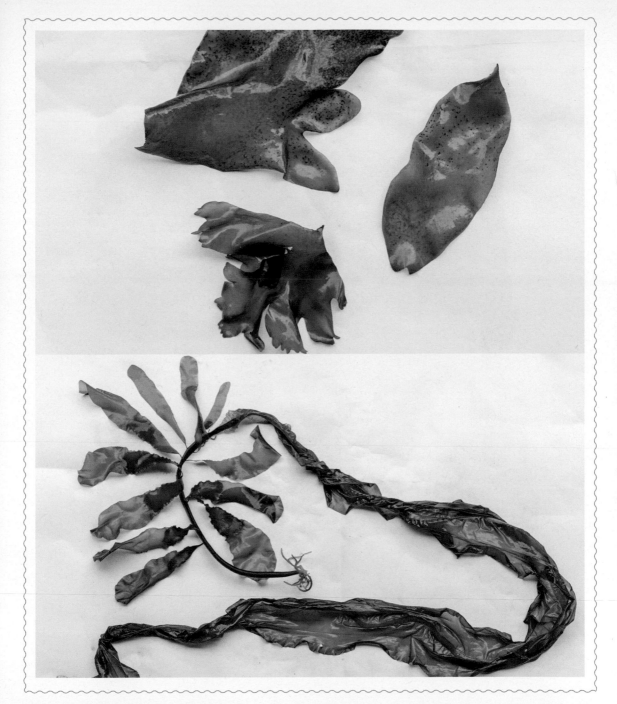

TOP: Dulse; BOTTOM: Winged Kelp

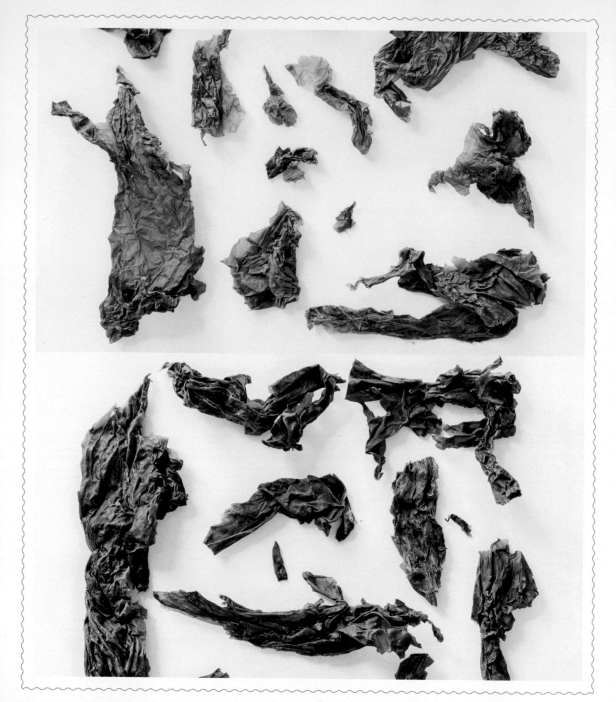

TOP: Dried Sea Lettuce; BOTTOM: Nori

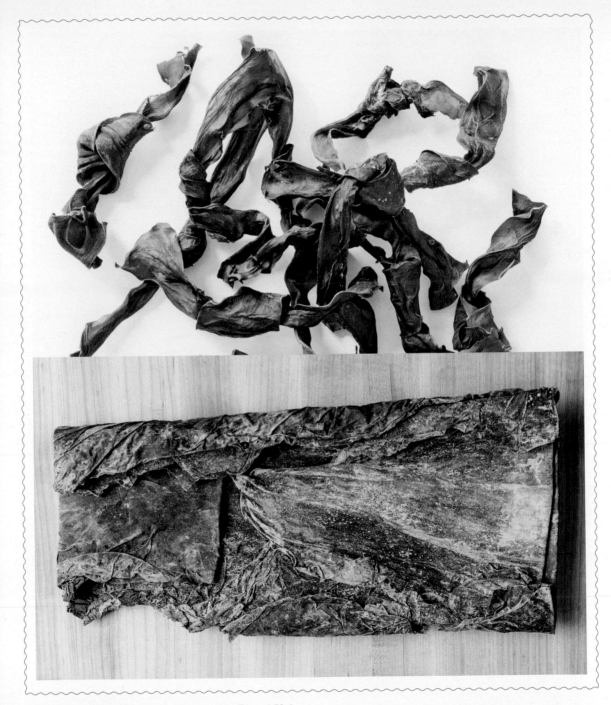

TOP: Dried Pacific Wakame; BOTTOM: Dried Kelp

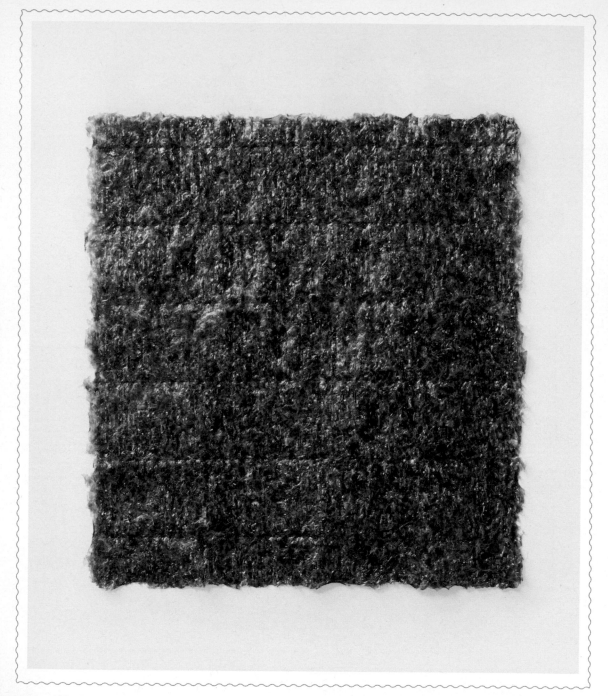

Nori Sheet

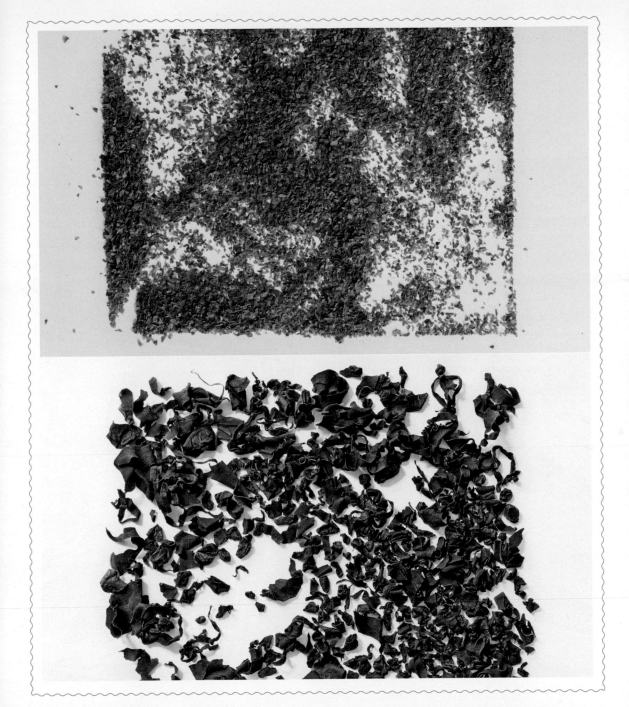

TOP: Sea Lettuce Flakes: BOTTOM: Nori

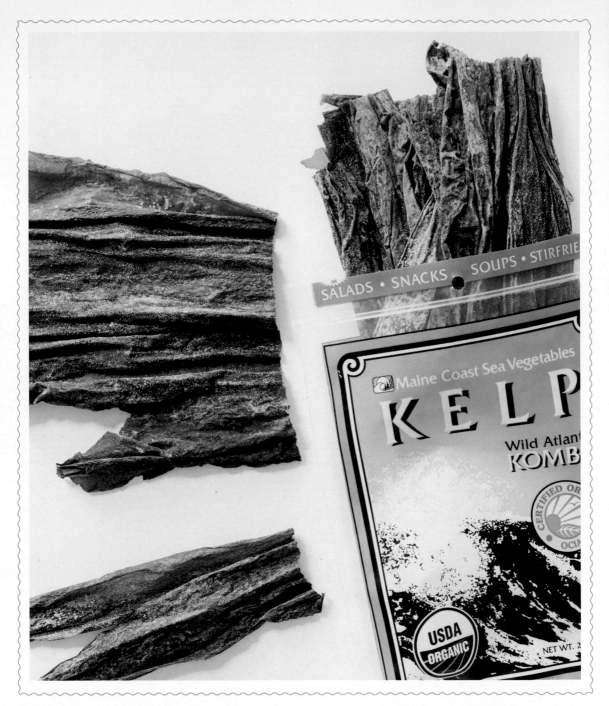

Packaged Dried Kelp

from different regions distinct characteristics, but once these salts are incorporated into a dish with many other flavors, those subtle nuances are lost. A coarse sel gris, or gray salt, is often the least expensive of the sea salts. Fleur de sel, a wind-evaporated, flowerlike crystal that forms on the surface of salt ponds, is often the most expensive. These salts all have their appeal but are often not worth the price when you are simply looking for a seasoning product.

• **FLAVORED SALTS** are combined with other seasonings: citrus zest, herbs, even wine. This book includes a few recipes for flavored salts, which are more similar to seasoning mixes. While these are certainly sexy on the store shelf, I recommend making them at home because the ingredients are often as simple as the name itself, and when made in small batches the flavors stay fresh and lively. It's best to make them in small batches as flavors can dull over time.

• **SMOKED SALT** is made with many different types of salt that are smoked using a number of different woods. Common flavors include applewood and hickory. They are often attractively rusty hued in tone and highly aromatic, and they can add a delightful punch of flavor into any dish they are incorporated into. Using smoked salt is effective in delivering a smoky backbone of flavor.

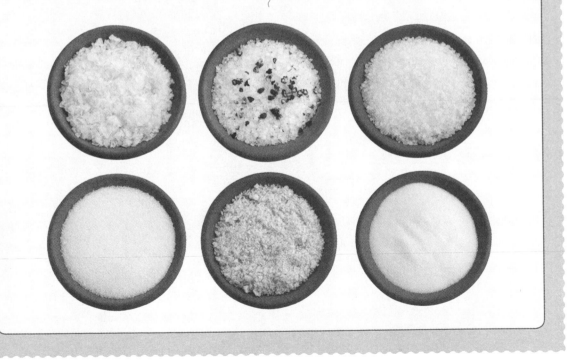

BUTTERNUT SQUASH AND SEAGREEN CAPONATA

SERVES 6–8

Caponata is a traditional southern Italian stew of vegetables, known for its sweet-sour personality. Here the sweet squash and onion melt into a lightly spiced and aromatic stew with peppers and fennel. The umami-rich seagreens add a third, charismatic dimension to the dish.

You can use fresh, frozen, or dried seagreens of any kind in this recipe. If you use fresh seagreens, it's best to add them at the end of the cooking time, so they don't break down too much. If you decide to use dried seagreens, be sure to add them at the beginning.

6   *tablespoons olive oil*

4   *tablespoons slivered almonds*

1   *ounce dried kelp or dulse (applewood-smoked is best)*

2   *stalks celery, cut into 1-inch pieces*

1   *bulb fennel, stalks discarded, cut into roughly 1-inch dice*

1   *large onion, cut into roughly 1-inch dice*

1   *medium-hot pepper, such as poblano, Anaheim, or Hungarian, seeded and cut into small dice*

1   *(2 ounce) can oil-packed anchovies*

1   *butternut squash, peeled and cut into roughly 1-inch cubes*

2   *(14 ounce) cans fire-roasted diced tomatoes*

2   *tablespoons molasses or maple syrup*

3   *tablespoons red wine vinegar*

    Juice of 1 lemon

    Kosher salt

1   *cup water*

3   *tablespoons chopped cilantro or parsley*

1. In a wide stew pot, heat the oil over high heat. Add the almonds and dried seagreens and cook until they are lightly toasted, about 3–4 minutes.

2. Add the celery, fennel, onion, and pepper. Sauté for another 5 minutes.

3. Add the anchovies with all of their oil. Mash the fillets into the oil until they dissolve.

4. Add the squash and toss to combine. Reduce the heat to medium and cook for 5 minutes.

5. Add the canned tomatoes, molasses or maple syrup, vinegar, and lemon juice. Season generously with salt. Stir to combine and cook until the tomatoes begin to break down and release their juices, about 10 minutes.

6. Add the water, stir to combine, and reduce the heat to low. Cover the pot and cook until the vegetables are soft but not falling apart, about 30 minutes.

7. Toss in the cilantro or parsley. Check the seasoning and adjust if necessary. This stew tastes best if you allow it to cool overnight. Reheat the stew over low heat before serving it the next day.

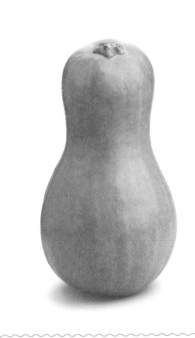

SAUTÉED SEAGREENS WITH BACON, APPLE, AND ONION

SERVES 4

Do you need an incentive to get someone in your life to try seagreens? Just add bacon!

- 4   *strips bacon*
- 2   *small onions, cut into wedges*
- 1   *apple, such as Pink Lady, cut into thin wedges*
- 1   *pound fresh or frozen sugar kelp, blanched and cut into bite-size pieces*
-     *Salt*

1. In a large sauté pan, brown the bacon and onion together. When the bacon is mostly crisp, pour off most of the fat.

2. Add the apple, toss to combine, and cook 2–3 minutes.

3. Add the seagreens and mix well. Cook until warmed through. Check the seasoning and adjust with salt, if needed.

BROILED CAULIFLOWER WITH MINT, SEAGREENS, AND PARMESAN

SERVES 4–6

This recipe is adapted from one of my earlier books, *Where There's Smoke* (Sterling Epicure, 2013). Here, broiled, lightly browned cauliflower is reinvigorated with aromatic mint and the crunch of seagreens. The Parmesan adds a beautiful twist and a lovely presentation.

1   *large head cauliflower*
    Kosher salt
8   *tablespoons extra virgin olive oil*
10 *sprigs fresh mint, leaves only, torn*
5   *tablespoons crumbled wakame or 5 sheets oven-crisped nori*
3   *tablespoons olive oil*
2   *ounces Parmesan cheese, shaved with a vegetable peeler*

1. Place the whole head of cauliflower in a large pot and cover it with cold water.

2. Season generously with salt and place over high heat.

3. Bring to a boil, then turn off the heat and let sit for 10 minutes. The cauliflower should be tender all the way through when pierced with a knife.

4. Gently remove the cauliflower, set it upside down on kitchen towels, and let it drain fully.

5. Drizzle the cauliflower with 5 tablespoons olive oil and place it with the floret side up under the broiler. Cook until the florets begin to caramelize, about 15 minutes.

6. Remove from the broiler and transfer the cauliflower to a serving platter. Garnish with mint and crumbled or crisped seagreens and drizzle with the remaining 3 tablespoons of olive oil.

7. Top with the Parmesan cheese and serve immediately. This dish is best served as a whole head so that people can easily spoon off sections at the table.

CRISPY ZUCCHINI CAKES WITH KELP AND CASHEW PESTO

SERVES 4

When summer strikes and zucchini is in full bloom, those of you with gardens know it can be challenging to keep up with the amount of food a single vine can produce. This dish is a great way to use your garden bounty—or take advantage of super-low pricing at your local grocery store or farmers' market at the height of the zucchini harvest.

1½ pounds zucchini, ends trimmed

    Kosher salt

½ pound finely chopped fresh or frozen kelp, squeezed as dry as possible

2 tablespoons plain Greek yogurt or labneh

¾ cup panko bread crumbs

¼ cup extra virgin olive oil, plus more if needed

1 recipe Kelp and Cashew Pesto (see page 80)

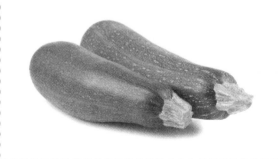

1. Shred the zucchini using the largest holes of a box grater, season it generously with salt, and put it into a colander set over a bowl. Let the zucchini sit for at least 4 hours and as long as overnight. You might be a little surprised at how much liquid comes out!

2. After it has drained, take a small quantity of the zucchini in your hand and squeeze it to extract as much liquid as possible; then place it in a second bowl. Repeat with all the zucchini.

3. Mix the zucchini with the kelp, yogurt, and bread crumbs. Toss to combine and let the mixture sit for at least 20 minutes so the crumbs have time to absorb any excess liquid. Form the mixture into small patties 2–3 inches in diameter.

4. In a large skillet, heat the olive oil over medium-high heat. When the oil is shimmering, add a few of the zucchini cakes at a time, cooking them until they are golden brown. Flip the cakes to cook on the other side, then remove them from the pan and keep them warm while you cook the remaining cakes, adding more oil to the pan if necessary.

5. Serve hot with a generous swoosh of the pesto.

POLENTA WITH SEAGREENS AND PARMESAN

SERVES 4

Polenta is cornmeal that has been simmered in liquid until it is soft and has a pudding-like texture. This makes for a heartwarming meal in the cold of winter, garnished with a warm salad of seagreens and flecked with Parmesan.

- 5 *cups of boiling water*
- 2 *ounces dried applewood-smoked dulse (or regular dulse)*
- 1 *cup medium- or coarse-ground cornmeal*
- 4 *tablespoons olive oil*
- 1 *clove garlic*
- 1 *cup room-temperature water*
- 2 *ounces Parmesan cheese, grated*

1. Pour the boiling water over the dulse and let it sit for 15 minutes. Strain the dulse, reserving the liquid, and put the dulse to the side. Measure the liquid and add water, as necessary, to make 5 full cups. Bring the liquid to a boil in a medium-sized heavy pot.

2. Pour the cornmeal into the liquid, stirring vigorously with a whisk. Continue stirring until the mixture begins to slightly thicken, about 4–5 minutes.

3. Turn the heat to low and cook about 1 hour, stirring two or three times throughout the cooking time. If the mixture becomes too thick, add water until the grains have completely softened and the texture is creamy. (If using instant polenta follow cooking times on package.)

4. Whisk in 2 tablespoons of the oil and let the mixture sit for 10 minutes.

5. To prepare the dulse, heat the remaining oil and garlic in a sauté pan over medium heat. Cook the garlic until it is golden brown.

6. Add the dulse and cook another 2 minutes, stirring to mix well. Add 1 cup of water and simmer until the dulse is rehydrated, about 3–5 minutes.

7. Serve the polenta in large bowls with a nest of dulse in the center of each bowl. Sprinkle with Parmesan and serve immediately.

UMAMI-RICH RICE PILAF

SERVES 4

Rice pilaf is an easy addition to any weeknight meal. Here, kelp lends beautiful flakes of color and textural contrast. Furikake adds a nice crunch, if you choose to use it, and almonds add a simple and easy nutritional boost.

- ¼ *ounce dried kelp (not rehydrated)*
- 3 *cups water*
- 5 *tablespoons extra virgin olive oil*
- 8 *ounces skinless almond slivers*

1 large bulb fennel, finely diced

2 cloves garlic, thinly sliced

1½ cups basmati or jasmine brown rice

Salt

Furikake for garnish, if desired (see page 70)

1. Simmer the kelp in the water for 7 minutes; reserve both.

2. Finely chop the kelp.

3. Heat the olive oil in a medium saucepan over medium-high heat and cook the almond slices until they are golden brown and heavily aromatic.

4. Add the fennel and garlic, cooking until they begin to wilt, about 3 minutes.

5. Add the rice, toss to coat the grains in oil, and cook, stirring occasionally, until the majority of the rice takes on a variety of golds and browns and charcoal blacks (yes, burning a little bit is perfectly fine).

6. Add the kelp, water, and salt. Cover the pan and bring to a boil. As it comes to a boil, remove the cover and cook over low heat for another 5 minutes.

7. Remove from the heat and let it sit 5 minutes for the grains to regain their texture and absorb the last of the cooking liquid. Fluff the rice with a fork to release the steam and serve on a large platter. If using, top with furikake.

CREAMED SEAGREENS

SERVES 4–8

This dish is a perfect accompaniment to winter feasts or simple meals. Akin to creamed spinach, it makes a delicious side dish for a nice standing rib roast, roast turkey, or seafood.

1 large onion, sliced thin

2 tablespoons butter

2 teaspoons freshly grated mace

Zest of 1 lemon

2 pounds fresh seagreens, or 8 cups rehydrated seagreens

1 cup heavy cream or sour cream

Cayenne

Salt

1. Sauté the onion in butter over medium heat until barely wilted.

2. Add the mace and lemon zest, and cook until fragrant, 1 minute.

3. Add the seagreens and cook until warmed through.

4. Add the heavy cream or sour cream and cayenne. Season with salt.

5. Bring to a simmer and serve as you would creamed spinach, or place in a casserole dish and bake at 325°F until bubbling at the sides and lightly browned on top.

SEAGREENS BRAISED COLLARD STYLE WITH APPLE CIDER

SERVES 4–6

This dish plays on a Southern classic, and its flavors improve and meld over time. I recommend making these lovely braised greens at least a day before you intend to serve them. Just reheat the dish over very low heat, and it's good to go. The addition, at the table, of a fiery hot sauce of chile peppers soaked in vinegar is a must in my book. When you serve the greens, be generous with the cooking liquid, known as the pot likker, because it is equally as good as, if not better than, the greens themselves.

2   onions, sliced thin

3   garlic cloves

¼   cup extra virgin olive oil

1   tablespoon chile flakes

1   pound meaty ham hocks

4   cups hard cider or regular cider

2   bay leaves
    Salt

6   cups (about 2 pounds) fresh or frozen seagreens, cut into 1-inch ribbons (or 4 ounces dried seagreens rehydrated in 1–2 cups water to rehydrate them)

1. In a large pot, sauté the onions and garlic in oil until softened, approximately 5–7 minutes.

2. Add the chile flakes and toast for 1 minute.

3. Add the ham hocks, cider, and bay leaves. Season lightly with salt and bring to a boil. Reduce the heat to low, cover, and simmer until the ham hocks are tender, about 2 hours.

4. Remove the ham hocks and bay leaves, and add the seagreens. Simmer until soft (30–60 minutes, depending on which seagreens you use).

5. Return the chopped ham meat to the soup, heat through, and serve.

FREE RADICALS AND ANTIOXIDANTS

Free radicals are formed constantly during digestion and especially when people are exposed to radiation or smoke. Evidence suggests that free radical buildup may contribute to cancer, heart disease, and arthritis. Antioxidants are nutrients that can partially block damaging free radicals. There are potentially thousands of different substances that can act as antioxidants; the most prevalent include vitamin C, vitamin E, beta-carotene, and minerals like selenium and manganese, which are found in seagreens.

BRAISED RED CABBAGE WITH SEAGREENS

SERVES 4–6

Braised red cabbage is an incredibly beautiful and colorful dish. The key to its success is plenty of vinegar, which smooths out the sometimes rough edges of the cabbage. The addition of goat cheese elevates this humble dish to the focal point of a very elegant meal.

½ *ounce kombu or applewood-smoked dulse*

2 *cups water*

2 *onions, sliced thin*

1 *teaspoon grated fresh ginger*

4 *tablespoons butter*

1 *small head red cabbage, sliced thin*

   Salt

1 *cinnamon stick*

4 *tablespoons red wine vinegar*

3 *tablespoons molasses*

4 *ounces goat cheese*

1. Simmer the seagreens in the water for 5 minutes. Strain and reserve both seagreens and the liquid.

2. Sauté the onion and ginger in butter until wilted, 3–4 minutes.

3. Add the cabbage and seagreens, and toss to coat. Season with salt.

4. Add the cinnamon stick, vinegar, molasses, and reserved seagreen cooking liquid, and bring to a simmer. Cover and cook about 30–40 minutes until the cabbage is tender but not falling apart.

5. Strain the cabbage, reserving the liquid. Reduce the reserved liquid to a thick syrup.

6. Return the cabbage to the pot with the syrup, check for seasoning, and toss to coat. Add crumbled goat cheese and serve.

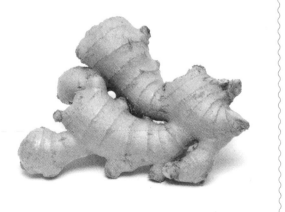

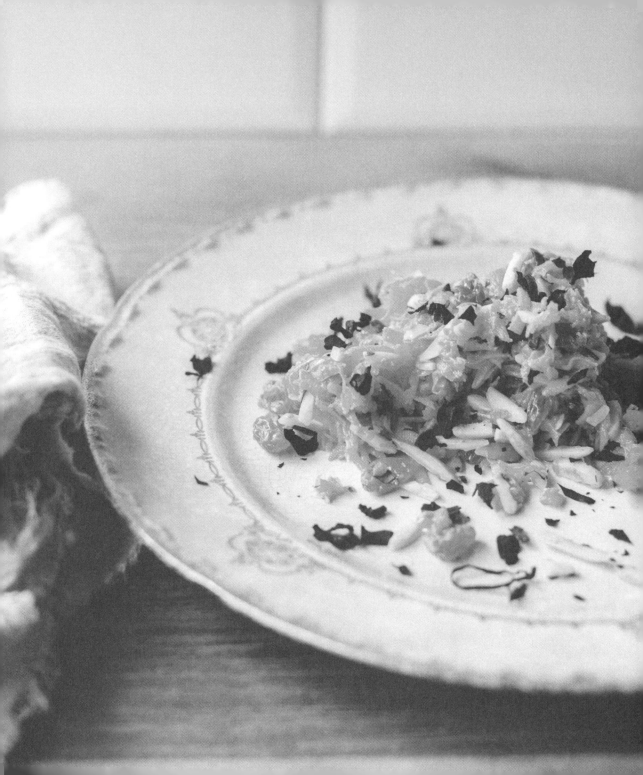

CHAPTER 9

SALADS

We often look to salads as a healthful meal and welcome the opportunity to plunder the local salad bar, piling one delicious flavor and texture on top of the next, combining it all into a one-of-a-kind dish. This flexible, creative outlook makes it easy to adapt seagreens to your salad-making habits. While the recipes here are more composed, I fully recommend simply adding seagreens to the regular flow of ingredients you use regularly. Try a little of this one day, a little of that the next. Top it all with kidney beans and your favorite vinaigrette, and you have a delightful meal.

Seagreens in salads are used in two very different ways. Fresh or frozen seagreens, such as sugar kelp and dulse, are used to add bulk. Dried seagreens, such as nori or wakame, are generally best used to add texture and flavor, whether whisked into vinaigrettes as powders or flakes, or crumbled on top as crunchy little bits. In either case, the salad will be all the better for it.

ARUGULA, MINT, APPLE, AND SEAGREENS SALAD

SERVES 4

The peppery bite and texture of arugula, the crunch of apple, the soaring aroma of mint, and the subtle saltiness of seagreens are an amazing combination. Get the sweetest apple you can find, such as Fuji or Braeburn.

3 tablespoons olive oil

1 tablespoon red wine vinegar

1 tablespoon whole grain or Dijon mustard
   Salt

½ pound arugula

½ pound fresh or frozen kelp cut into bite-size pieces, or 2 ounces rehydrated, dried kelp

2 crisp apples, such as Fuji or Braeburn, very thinly sliced

10 sprigs mint, leaves only, julienned
   Fresh cracked pepper

1. In a large bowl whisk together the olive oil, vinegar, mustard, and a good pinch of salt.

2. Add the arugula, seagreens, apple, and mint and toss until well coated. Serve immediately with fresh cracked pepper.

OPPOSITE: **Moroccan Salad, page 104**

SUMMER CORN SALAD

SERVES 4

Of all fresh salad ingredients, corn is accentuated the most by the addition of umami flavors in seagreens. Here the combination of slightly crunchy corn kernels and delightfully sweet ripe cherry tomatoes, heightened by fresh cilantro, makes for an easy to put together, easy to make ahead, easy to please salad.

6 *ears corn, shucked and boiled for 8 minutes in salted water*

1 *cup cherry tomatoes (Sun Gold is my favorite, though any variety will do; avoid pear tomatoes, as they can be mealy and tasteless)*

1 *small red onion, finely diced, then washed briefly under cold running water*

2 *tablespoons chopped fresh cilantro*

Juice of 2 limes

1 *tablespoon extra virgin olive oil*

Kosher salt

4 *sheets toasted nori, torn into small pieces*

1. Cut the cooked kernels from the corn cobs with a paring knife into a large bowl. Do not cut too deeply, or the base of the kernel will be tough—but don't go too shallow either, or you'll lose precious flavor.

2. After the kernels have been cut, scrape the cobs with the back of the knife to "milk" any remaining corn juice into the bowl.

3. Slice the tomatoes in half and combine them with the corn.

4. Add the onion, cilantro, lime juice, olive oil, and salt to taste. Toss to combine.

5. Taste for seasoning and adjust if necessary.

6. Top with torn nori. Serve at room temperature.

WATERMELON SALAD WITH LIME, MINT, AND NORI

SERVES 8–12

Watermelon is rarely thought of in the context of savory dishes, since it is usually eaten unadorned as a snack or light dessert. However, when watermelon is paired with fresh herbs, nori, and the bite of olive oil and chiles, it is transformed as a wonderfully savory-sweet salad ingredient. This recipe makes quite a bit of salad, as even the smallest watermelon yields quite a lot. Don't worry about having too much, however— it'll go fast.

8 *cups diced seedless watermelon (about 1 medium melon)*

¼ cup olive oil

1–2 teaspoons chile flakes

Juice of 2 limes

Salt

6 sprigs fresh mint, leaves only

8 sheets toasted nori, torn, or 1 cup wakame

1. In a large bowl, combine the watermelon, oil, chile flakes, and lime juice. Season to taste with salt.

2. Finely slice the mint leaves and toss to combine with the salad at the last minute before serving.

3. Top with torn nori or wakame. Do not serve this dish too cold, or the flavors will be muted.

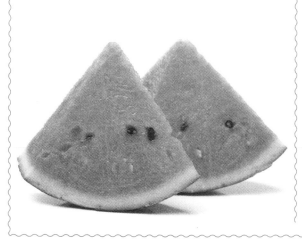

SEA-SMOKY MEDITERRANEAN SALAD

SERVES 4

The preparation of this salad requires nothing more than a little knife work. This salad is delightful as a meal by itself or paired with grilled or baked seafood served chilled.

2 tomatoes, sliced

1 red onion, sliced thinly and rinsed briefly under cold running water

1 green pepper, sliced as thin as possible

1 mild chile, such as Anaheim, sliced into rounds

Juice of 1 lime

1 tablespoon extra virgin olive oil

Salt

1 clove garlic, grated with a Microplane grater or finely diced

¼ ounce applewood-smoked dulse, crumbled and toasted

1. Toss the tomatoes, onion, green pepper, and chile together.

2. In a separate bowl combine the lime juice, olive oil, salt, garlic, and dulse.

3. Stir to combine, then toss with the vegetables. Let sit for at least 5 minutes before serving.

SPICY SMASHED CUCUMBER WITH CANDIED GINGER

SERVES 4

We often think of cucumbers only as sticks or slices, but cutting them into 1-inch rounds and then smashing them with a potato masher or the underside of a pot results in a variety of shapes and sizes as well as a coarser texture. Some of the pulp becomes a purée, helping to thicken the vinaigrette, and it makes for a fabulous presentation as well as a way to better flavor the cucumber throughout.

1   *large cucumber, cut into 1-inch sections and smashed*

1   *shallot, sliced into thin rings*

4   *sprigs mint leaves, finely sliced*

1   *tablespoon sesame oil*

2   *tablespoons rice wine vinegar*

½   *tablespoon soy sauce*

1   *tablespoon minced candied ginger or grated fresh*

2   *teaspoons chile flakes*

2   *tablespoons dulse flakes*

1. Toss all ingredients to combine. Let sit 5 minutes before serving at room temperature.

FENNEL, CARROT, AND SEAGREENS SALAD

SERVES 4

Carrots—not often thought of as an elegant ingredient—can be precisely that when peeled into long, thin, confetti-like strands. Simply use a peeler, rotating the carrot as you peel, and discarding the woody inner core. The earthiness of the carrot paired with herbaceous fennel and briny seagreens makes for an incredibly beautiful dish, as elegant as a first course as it is on a picnic blanket. Smoked seafood, such as trout, is a particularly wonderful addition to this salad.

1   *bulb fennel*

1   *red onion*

2   *carrots*

½   *pound fresh seagreens, blanched and shredded*

1   *cup cilantro leaves*

2   *tablespoons whole grain mustard*

1½ *tablespoons red wine vinegar*

4   *tablespoons extra virgin olive oil*

1   *teaspoon ground allspice*
    Salt

1. Thinly slice the fennel and red onion using a mandoline slicer.

FENNEL

If I had to choose one crop to grow on a desert island, it would be fennel. Fennel has an incredible, beguiling, and nuanced flavor that either can be coaxed into a pronounced and evocative presence in a dish, or can become an understated, elegant, and alluring component.

The fennel bulb, as commonly found in grocery stores, often comes with a few inches of the green stalks extending beyond the layered bulb. The stalks and their very tender frilly fronds—a lacy and delicate, beautiful thin leaf—are reminiscent of fine needlework. These fronds have a gentle and delicate flavor and little aroma, but their presence grows as you get further into the meal.

Similar to chervil in their use, fennel fronds must be added at the very end of the preparation, just prior to serving, or their texture will degrade as they wilt. The green stalks themselves can be quite fibrous and woody, similar to celery in their appearance, but fully round. The stalks must be sliced very thin in order to be effectively used. Much like the whites of scallions, these thin disks can add wonderful texture and an interesting and unexpected flavor to salads, especially vegetable salads that include cucumbers, tomato, feta cheese, and olives.

Fennel's perfect partner in this world is citrus. The mostly sweet, gently sour orange brings out the highest and best qualities of the anise-flavored fennel. A classic dish combines fennel and oranges with salty cured black olives, which, like some seagreens, lend not only a definitive briny punch but also an umami richness that broadens the overall flavor composition of the dish.

The fennel bulb itself can be used when sliced thin into disks and has a slightly more spicy flavor, more akin to a radish than to the delicate and aromatic outer leaves. Pairing fennel with seagreens cannot go wrong. Fennel has a cooling personality that is very similar to the most commonly used seagreens, and fennel's bulk is a good foil for their powerful flavors.

2. Using a peeler, make long, thin strips of the carrots, stopping when you reach the core.

3. Combine the fennel, onion, carrots, seagreens, and cilantro in a large bowl.

4. In a separate bowl, mix the mustard, vinegar, olive oil, allspice, and a generous portion of salt. Whisk to combine.

5. Mix the vinaigrette with the vegetables and toss to combine.

MOROCCAN SALAD

SERVES 4

When I was living in Morocco, a traditional salad of carrots sweetened with raisins and vinegar accompanied many meals. Here the addition of crispy wakame adds complexity, richness, and a crunch that contrasts interestingly with the carrot.

1 *pound carrots, finely shredded in a food processor or on a box grater*

½ *cup golden raisins*

½ *cup slivered almonds*

¼ *cup red wine vinegar*

¼ *cup cilantro, chopped*

½ *cup olive oil*

   Salt

1 *cup dried wakame*

1. Mix the carrots, raisins, almonds, vinegar, cilantro, and olive oil together and season with salt. Garnish with wakame and serve.

MODERN CUISINE

Alginic acid (alginato) is used in contemporary culinary techniques such as spherification (controlled "jellification" of a liquid in order to make spheres) made famous by chef and restaurateur Ferran Adrià.

CELERY ROOT SLAW WITH SEAGREENS

SERVES 4

All too often, when we think of slaw, only cabbage comes to mind. But celery root, the knobby, gnarly cousin of the green cabbage we know so well, has a soft texture and lingering crunch that makes it a perfect substitute for cabbage. The seagreens here add a wonderful contrast to the sweet, earthy flavor of the celery root.

¼ *cup sherry vinegar*

2 *teaspoons chile flakes*

⅔ *cup sour cream or Greek yogurt*
   Salt

1 *large celery root, peeled and cut into thin strips*

1 *red bell pepper, seeded and cut into thin strips*

2 *cups dried kombu, rehydrated in warm water and cut into thin strips*

1 *red onion, sliced thin and rinsed briefly in cold water*

1. Combine the vinegar, chile flakes, and sour cream in a large bowl. Season with salt and add the celery root, bell pepper, kombu, and onion. Toss to combine. Adjust the seasoning with salt if needed. Let the slaw sit at least 20 minutes before serving.

CRUNCHY QUINOA, SWEET POTATO, AND SEAGREENS

SERVES 4

What more is there to say? This recipe is loaded with superfoods. It can be made in big batches, save for the wakame garnish, which is best added just prior to serving. This is a fabulous dish to have on hand for lunch or dinner, or to snack on throughout the week.

1   sweet potato, peeled and cut into roughly
    ½-inch cubes

2–3 cups Basic Dashi Broth (see page 111,
    or use store-bought broth)

1   cup quinoa, washed under cold running
    water

⅓   cup slivered almonds

½   bunch mint, leaves picked and torn

⅓   cup raisins

    Salt

¼   cup dried wakame

1. Cook the sweet potato in seasoned broth until soft. Remove the sweet potato and reserve both the sweet potato and broth.

2. Add enough broth to make 2 cups, add quinoa, and cook until soft. Drain the quinoa and let air dry for 10 minutes.

QUINOA

Although it is considered a grain, much like amaranth, this is actually the seed of a plant that grows in arid conditions. The sacred food of the Incan empire, quinoa is indigenous to the northern countries of South America. Quinoa cooks like any other grain. Prior to use, however, quinoa should be rinsed thoroughly under cold running water, as there is typically a powdery resin on the seeds that becomes quite bitter when cooked. Rinsing removes this, leaving the flavor sweet and nutty.

3. Toss the quinoa with the slivered almonds, mint, and raisins. Fold in the sweet potato and combine.

4. Season with salt. Top with dried wakame.

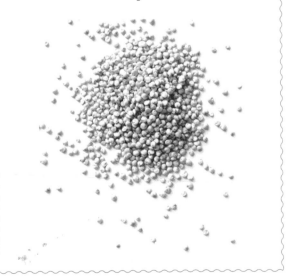

COASTAL QUINOA TABBOULEH

SERVES 4

Tabbouleh, soaked bulgur wheat, is already a powerhouse of nutrition and energy, and when paired with near equal amounts of parsley, the flavorful result is truly winning. The freshness of this salad is further punctuated with diced tomato. In this recipe, trade out as much of the parsley as you care to with seagreens, even using a mixture of different seagreens to suit your taste.

- 1 cup quinoa, washed under cold running water
- 2 cups water
- ¼ cup mint leaves, finely sliced
- ½ cup parsley, finely chopped
- ½ cup bulgur, soaked for 1 hour or more in ½ cup vinegar and 1 cup water
- 1 plum tomato, finely diced
- 1 pound fresh or frozen seagreens, blanched, rinsed, and finely chopped, or 2 ounces dried kombu, rehydrated*
- ¼ cup olive oil
- ¼ cup red wine vinegar
   Salt

1. Boil quinoa in 2 cups of water for 15 minutes. Allow to rest off the heat for 15 minutes. Fluff with fork and chill.

2. Combine the chilled quinoa with the mint, parsley, bulgur, tomato, and seagreens. Dress with olive oil and red wine vinegar. Season with salt and let sit 1 hour before serving.

* If using dried kombu, use 2 cups of the rehydrating liquid to cook the quinoa. (See page 120.)

PEAR AND HERBS OVER SEAGREENS SALAD

SERVES 4

Although this recipe calls for kelp, any number of seagreens will do—fresh or rehydrated dried seagreens will work equally well. Fresh or frozen kelp, as a wet green, provides the nicest contrast in texture; however, dried wakame or dulse that has been toasted in the oven is a wonderful textural pairing.

- 4 pears, cut into ½-inch wedges
- 1 bunch mint, leaves only, finely sliced
- ¼ cup red wine vinegar
- 2 stalks celery, shaved thin
- 2 shallots, shaved thin, rinsed under cold running water for 1 minute
- 6 cups kelp, blanched and cut into bite-size pieces, or 2 ounces dried kelp, rehydrated
- ½ cup olive oil
   Salt

1. Combine all ingredients. Let marinate for 20 minutes prior to serving.

BEET AND SEAGREEN SALAD

SERVES 4

Beets and walnuts are a perfect combination that is full of nutrition, and the addition of seagreens brings a welcome flavor contrast to the earthy beets. When the walnuts are toasted, this dish really sings.

3 *large beets*

½ *pound fresh or frozen sugar kelp cut into bite-size pieces, or 1 ounce dried kombu, rehydrated and sliced**

   Juice of ½ lemon

¼ *cup walnut oil (optional)*

¼ *cup olive oil (if not using walnut oil, simply double the olive oil)*

   Salt

⅓ *cup walnut pieces*

1. Boil the beets in salted water until soft. Peel and dice them into 1-inch pieces.

2. Combine the beets and kelp. Season with lemon juice, walnut oil, and olive oil, and season with salt. Crumble the walnut pieces over the top and serve.

* If using dried kombu, cook the beets in the rehydrating liquid with added water if necessary.

SEASHORE PANZANELLA

SERVES 4

Panzanella is a very interesting combination of ingredients, in that much of the structure and crunch comes from the inclusion of chips or croutons, traditionally made from day-old bread. I like to use pita chips, as they combine well with other ingredients and allow for better integration of flavors.

1 *small butternut squash, peeled and cut into 1-inch dice*

¼ *cup olive oil*

3 *cups red seedless grapes, cut in half*

1 *ounce dried kombu, rehydrated and cut into bite-size pieces*

3 *tablespoons red wine vinegar*

   Salt

¼ *cup walnut pieces*

2 *cups pita chips, crumbled*

1. Preheat the oven to 425°F. Toss the squash with 2 tablespoons of the olive oil and roast until soft. Remove from the oven and let cool.

2. Toss the grapes and kombu with the vinegar and remaining olive oil, and season with salt. Let sit 5 minutes.

3. Add the butternut squash, walnuts, and pita chips and toss. Adjust the seasoning as needed and let sit 15 minutes before serving.

SEAGREENS SUSHI JOINT–STYLE SALAD

SERVES 4

This is a fresh take on the classic neon-green sushi restaurant offering. You'd be surprised how balanced this dish can be when made with fresh, high-quality ingredients. It can be left to marinate up to 2 days; however, the fresh herbs should be added just prior to serving.

- 1½ tablespoons rice vinegar
- 1 tablespoon aji-mirin (sweet rice wine)
- ½ tablespoon toasted sesame oil
- 1 tablespoon soy sauce
- ½ teaspoon salt
- ¼ teaspoon ground ginger
- ½ teaspoon garlic powder
- ½ chile pepper, such as serrano or Fresno, sliced super fine
- 1 ounce dried kombu, rehydrated, drained, and cut into very thin strips
- 1 ounce dried wakame
- 1 tablespoon toasted sesame seeds
- 4 scallions, finely chopped

CHILES

With few exceptions, seagreens pair beautifully with soft spice. While some seagreens are certainly very outgoing and prominent in any dish, most seagreens benefit from pairing with ingredients that complement their subtle and nuanced flavors. In my opinion, of all the ingredients that flatter seagreens, chiles are tops. Overly spicy chiles can be simply overwhelming, not just to seagreens but to all foods. I prefer to use fresh chiles, as the texture and slight fruitiness is most complementary. I most prefer peppers that lean toward sweet but still carry just a whisper of personality and a gentle kick. Among my favorites are Fresno and serrano. Sliced super thin or diced into a fine mince, the chiles add a slight crunch of texture that blends seamlessly into a dish. Basic crushed red chile flakes are a great addition, though powdered chile varieties, such as Espellete, peri peri, and Aleppo, are preferable. Another application of heat as a means to bloom the personality of seagreens is the incredibly elegant and stylish chipotle in adobo. A smoked jalapeño pepper stewed in spices into a rich paste, chipotle adds an incredible depth and complexity of flavor. Smoke is a complementary addition to many seagreens, and the added personality of the warm flavors of caramelized tomato and baking spices provide an excellent contrast to the cool character of seagreens.

1. Combine the rice vinegar, aji-mirin, sesame oil, soy sauce, salt, ginger, garlic powder, and chiles to make a dressing.

2. Toss with the seagreens and let marinate for at least 1 hour.

3. Before serving, top with sesame seeds and scallion.

KELP, TURNIP, AND SWEET ONION SALAD

SERVES 4

Here, smooth-flavored kelp is well matched with the spitfire bite of raw turnip. The sweet onion steps in to make sure everything stays well balanced.

1   *pound fresh or frozen kelp, torn in bite-size pieces, or 2 ounces dried kelp, rehydrated*

1   *Vidalia onion, sliced razor thin or shaved finely*

4   *small turnips, peeled and sliced thin*

½   *bunch flat-leaf parsley, leaves only*

2   *tablespoons sesame oil*

2   *tablespoons olive oil*

1   *orange, juiced*

2   *tablespoons balsamic vinegar*
    Salt

1. Mix all ingredients and toss to combine. Let sit 10 minutes before serving.

SEAGREENS WITH ITALIAN FENNEL SALAD

SERVES 4

The peppery bite of radish and the salty tang of olives pair incredibly well with the sweet coolness of oranges in this recipe. Throw in some sea-breeze-scented seagreens, and this classic combination is ready to be reintroduced.

½   *pound radishes, thinly sliced*

1   *bulb fennel, thinly sliced*

2   *cups fresh or frozen sugar kelp, blanched, or 1 ounce rehydrated, cut into bite-size pieces*

¼   *cup yellow raisins*

¼   *cup Kalamata olives, pitted and sliced*

4   *oranges, peeled and cut into segments*

3   *tablespoons red wine vinegar*
    Salt

3   *tablespoons olive oil*

1. Mix all ingredients and toss to combine. Let sit for 30 minutes before serving.

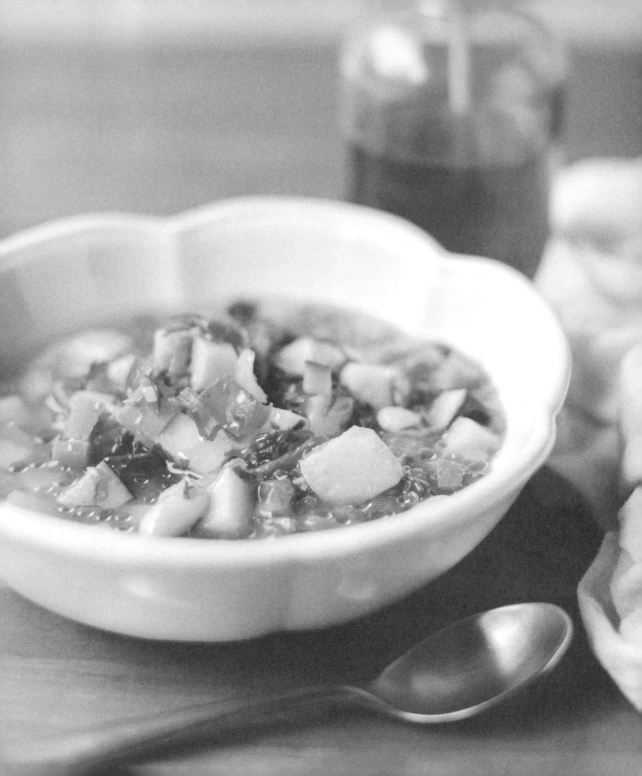

CHAPTER 10

SOUPS

Soups are probably the easiest way to introduce seagreens into your everyday cooking. In the United States, simple seagreen broth has long been enjoyed in the form of miso soup, although few of us have ever considered it a seagreens dish. In each of the recipes that follow, seagreen flavor is used to coax even more personality from traditional soup ingredients, while the whole is brought into focus through the addition of acid. In fact, I recommend spiking any soup you make with a bit of vinegar as a means of really bringing the flavors into focus. In fact, I recommend spiking any soup you make with a bit of acid.

BROTHS

Broths are one of the most fundamental ways to introduce flavor and to carry it throughout a dish. They are of course a base for soups, although they can also be used to make everything from risottos to pasta dishes. Broths are superb poaching liquids for seafood or chicken. I greatly enjoy them as restoratives, sipping them hot from a mug on a cold winter's day.

These recipes make enough for 2 uses, the extra freezes well, though the quantities of the recipes can easily be halved.

BASIC DASHI BROTH
MAKES 1 GALLON

- 1 gallon water
- 2 ounces shredded dried kelp or nori
- ¼ cup bonito flakes

1. Bring the water and shredded seagreens to a gentle simmer in a 6-quart saucepan. After 20 minutes, remove the greens with a slotted spoon and reserve them for another use.

2. Add the bonito flakes. As soon as the broth returns to a gentle simmer, remove the pan from the heat and strain.

3. Chill up to 4 days or freeze up to 1 month.

OPPOSITE: **Minestrone Soup, page 117**

BONITO FLAKES

One of the principal ingredients of the Japanese soup stock called dashi is a dried and flaked fish called skipjack, which is a kind of tuna, also known as bonito. These fish fillets are salted and often smoked, fermented, and dried until they can be shaved into razor-thin flakes. Adding these flakes to stock in the last few minutes of cooking gives it an incredible richness and depth of flavor that balances out the vegetal qualities of seagreens with a pleasant seafood flavor. The addition of bonito flakes does not add a strong flavor to a dish; rather, it complements and rounds it out, giving it an undercurrent of complexity.

AROMATIC DASHI BROTH

MAKES 1 GALLON

- 1 cup white wine
- 2 star anise pods
- 2 strips lemon peel
- 2 slices fresh ginger
- 1 gallon water
- 2 ounces shredded dried kelp or nori, dry toasted
- ¼ cup bonito flakes

1. In a 6-quart pot, boil the wine, star anise, lemon peel, and ginger until the wine cooks off. Add the water and shredded seagreens and reduce the heat to a gentle simmer. After 20 minutes, remove the greens with a slotted spoon and reserve them for another use.

2. Add the bonito flakes. As soon as the broth returns to a gentle simmer, remove the pan from heat and strain. Do not boil for long, as the goal is to keep the broth light and sharp and clear in flavor. If boiled, the stock will become murky and lose its focused flavor. Chill up to 4 days or freeze up to 1 month.

3. Use this as a stock as is or finish with lemon and herbs and serve as a consommé-like dish. Also try adding mace, dried or fresh chiles, onion, fennel, or fennel seeds to the cooking process to add depth of flavor.

VEGETABLE AND SEAGREEN BROTH

MAKES 1 GALLON

- 1 gallon water
- 1 onion, peeled and sliced
- 1 stalk celery
- 2 ounces dried kelp or nori
- 2 slices fresh ginger
- ½ cup dried mushrooms, preferably shiitake

1. Bring all ingredients to a gentle simmer in a 6-quart saucepan. Lower the heat and simmer for 20 minutes.

2. Remove from the heat and allow to steep for 1 hour. Strain out and discard the solids.

3. Chill up to 4 days or freeze in ice cube trays up to 1 month.

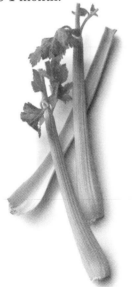

CHICKEN AND SEAGREEN STOCK

MAKES 1 GALLON

- 1 small chicken (about 2 pounds), skin removed and chopped into pieces
- 1 onion, peeled and sliced
- 1 carrot, peeled and chopped
- 1 stalk celery
- 5 quarts water
   Salt
- 5 allspice berries
- 1 star anise pod
- 2 ounces dried kelp or nori
- 1 lemon, cut in half

1. Add the chicken, onion, carrot, and celery to a 6-quart saucepan. Cover with water. Season generously with salt. Gradually heat over low heat until the liquid is steaming.

2. Add the allspice and anise. Cover the pot and simmer on low heat for 3–4 hours.

3. Add the seagreens and simmer another 10 minutes. Turn off the heat, add the lemon halves, and let steep for 30 minutes, then strain and discard the vegetables.

4. Reserve the seagreens and chicken meat for another use.

SOUPS

GAZPACHO

SERVES 4–6

Gazpacho is one of those dishes that you can make out of almost any vegetable. It's really meant to be a simple purée of whatever seasonal ingredients are freshest and best. It can be a deliciously fresh summer soup or even a combination of raw and boiled ingredients for a heartier, room temperature butternut squash version in the fall. Any way you make it, the key combination to gazpacho is bell peppers, onion, garlic, and cucumber as the backbone and either puréed squash or tomatoes as a basic flavoring. I like to garnish gazpacho with smoked seafood, especially mussels and clams, but crumbled hot-smoked salmon is also a delight.

1   cucumber, peeled and roughly chopped

1   small yellow onion, roughly chopped

1   red bell pepper, seeds removed and chopped

3   large ripe tomatoes, roughly chopped, or 2 (14 ounce) cans fire-roasted diced tomatoes

1   clove garlic, peeled

½   bunch cilantro or parsley

1   ounce dried applewood-smoked dulse or kelp

2   cups water

4   tablespoons red wine vinegar
    Salt

¼   cup extra virgin olive oil

1. Combine the cucumber, onion, red pepper, tomatoes, garlic, cilantro or parsley, seagreens, water, and vinegar in a food processor and process until you have a superfine texture.

2. Remove to a bowl, season with salt, and chill for at least 1 hour, up to 1 day.

3. Just prior to serving, whisk in the olive oil and adjust the seasoning if necessary.

GARLIC

Nearly universal in its application in global cuisines, garlic can provide a heady kick to dishes when added in its raw form, though this can be mitigated by grating just before use on a Microplane grater. When sautéed, it looses a lot of its bite and gains a soft nuttiness. This can be quite flattering to seagreens, giving them a nice, earthy, aromatic sweetness that draws out some of the their most charming qualities. Garlic is especially good in sautéed dishes or salads where seagreens are treated with a heavily flavored vinaigrette.

CALDO (SEA) VERDE

SERVES 4–6

This dish takes its inspiration from the classic Portuguese dish caldo verde, a workingman's meal packed with energy and calories to last all day. The potatoes are traditionally simmered until they completely break down and form a rich purée. In this version of caldo verde, the flavor of seagreens courses through the entire dish, adding a very pleasant color and texture. The soup can be made even more hearty and elegant with the addition of a spicy sausage, such as linguiça or chorizo, but my favorite thing to add is a can of smoked mussels or clams, allowing them to steep in the soup for a few minutes before serving.

4   *tablespoons olive oil*

1   *onion, minced*

1   *clove garlic, minced*

4   *russet potatoes, peeled and roughly chopped*

2   *quarts water or Vegetable and Seagreen Broth (see page 113)*

    Salt

    Ground black pepper

1   *pound fresh or frozen seagreens, rinsed and julienned, or 2 ounces dried seagreens (not rehydrated)*

1   *(6 ounce) can smoked mussels (optional)*

1. In a large saucepan, heat 3 tablespoons of the olive oil over medium heat. Add the onion and garlic and cook for 3 minutes.

2. Stir in the potatoes and cook for a few minutes until they begin to soften.

3. Add the water or broth, season with salt and pepper, and bring to a boil. Simmer for 20 minutes, until the potatoes begin to fall apart.

4. Mash the potatoes in the saucepan with a wooden spoon.

5. Stir in the seagreens. Cover and simmer 5 minutes, until the seagreens are tender and deep green.

6. Add the mussels and stir to warm.

7. Finish with the remaining olive oil and adjust seasoning if needed. Serve immediately.

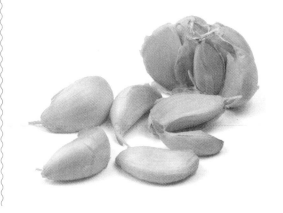

BEANS

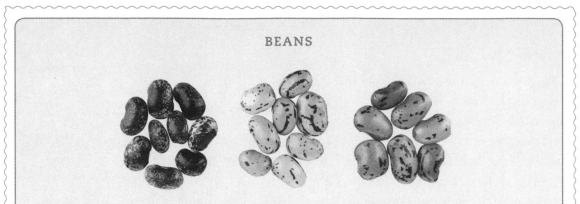

Although beans come in a common shape, that's where the similarities stop. Ranging from the glowing white cannellini or navy bean to the deep, staining hue of the black bean, just about every color and pattern is represented somewhere in between. Beans have very different flavors, especially with the recent reintroduction of heritage varieties such as Jacob's cattle, Dragon Tongue, cranberry, and rattlesnake, to list just a few of the delightfully named varieties. Each of these has a flavor all its own, although any one of them can pretty much stand in for the other. The cooking time and method for preparing beans is almost identical regardless of the variety. And of course beans across many varieties provide fiber, protein, manganese, iron, potassium, zinc, and other healthy phytonutrients.

SOAKING BEANS

• To cook dry beans most efficiently, it's best to soak them in cold water overnight, if you have the time, or give them a quick soak by pouring boiling water over them, letting them soak for 1 hour, then draining them before cooking. There is a theory that adding seagreens to beans hastens the cooking time. I'm not sure about that, but I do know that it makes them taste better.

RINSING CANNED BEANS

• Though many purists will tell you that cooking dried beans from scratch is the only way to go, I think that canned beans are a perfectly good ingredient. Though the varieties available are fewer than heritage dried beans, the ease and convenience of use makes it far more likely that they will find their way into an everyday meal. Canned beans should be rinsed prior to use, as the accompanying starchy liquid that surrounds them can bring tinny qualities to dishes and in some cases an unpleasant color. One drawback of canned beans is they tend to be very high in sodium, but washing helps to minimize this.

LENTIL SOUP

SERVES 4–6

This hearty soup is enjoyed equally well hot or cold, as a hearty meal for a summer luncheon or a warm winter restorative. The marriage of dulse and lentils is perfect, and the flavors meld seamlessly. The key to this soup is a little bit of smoke. To impart that flavor, I use smoked sweet paprika. Applewood-smoked dulse, however, would work just as well.

3 *tablespoons olive oil*

1 *onion, finely diced*

1 *tablespoon smoked sweet paprika*

¼ *cup dulse flakes*

3 *cups brown lentils, soaked in cold water for 2 hours, then drained*

6 *cups vegetable broth, dashi, or chicken stock*

1 *sprig thyme*

   Bay leaf

   Salt

1. In the olive oil, sauté the onion until it is translucent, about 5 minutes. Add the paprika and dulse, stir to combine, and cook 1 minute.

2. Add the lentils, broth, thyme, and bay leaf. Simmer for 20–40 minutes until the lentils are soft but not falling apart. Season with salt as needed. This soup is best chilled and served reheated or cold.

MINESTRONE

SERVES 4–6

This classic soup, a combination of just about anything that's available, is even easier to make in this version, because the seagreens are cooked into the broth along with the other ingredients, thus reducing overall cooking time. While this recipe calls for specific ingredients, ultimately a minestrone is just a vehicle for your own favorite ingredients.

6 *cups water*

½ *ounce dulse flakes or 1 ounce dried kelp*

1 *(14 ounce) can cannellini beans, drained and rinsed*

3 *carrots, peeled and medium diced*

4 *tomatoes, diced*

1 *bunch scallions, sliced thin*

1 *bay leaf*

1 *celery root, peeled and medium diced (substitute 2 russet potatoes if desired)*

2 *parsnips, peeled and medium diced*

1 *zucchini, medium diced*

   Salt

6 *tablespoons extra virgin olive oil*

1. In a large pot add the water, seagreens, beans, carrots, tomatoes, scallions, bay leaf, celery root, and parsnips. Bring to a low

(continued)

simmer and cook until the carrots are just soft, about 30 minutes.

2. Remove the bay leaf, add the zucchini, and season with salt. Simmer for 10 minutes, then remove from the heat.

3. Add the olive oil and serve immediately.

SHELLING BEAN SOUP

SERVES 4–6

It's believed that cooking dry beans with seagreens not only helps digestion but also speeds the cooking process, softening the beans more effectively. I don't know whether this is true or not because ever since I started cooking beans with seagreens, I haven't seen any reason to do it any other way.

3   *tablespoons butter*

½   *pound tasso or bacon, cubed*

3   *celery stalks, sliced*

3   *carrots, peeled and diced*

1   *leek, sliced*

½   *red onion, diced*

2   *garlic cloves, sliced*

1   *cup dried beans, such as kidney, cannellini, or cranberry, soaked overnight*

1   *bay leaf*

1   *chile pepper, such as serrano or Fresno*

1   *ounce dried kombu or ½ ounce dried dulse flakes*

6   *cups seagreen stock (see pages 111–113) or water*

Salt

1. In the butter, sauté the tasso or bacon until well colored. Add the celery, carrots, leek, onion, and garlic and cook for 1 minute. Add the beans, bay leaf, chile, and seagreens. Add the stock or water and bring to a simmer. Cover the pot and cook over low heat until the beans begin to soften, approximately 1 hour. Uncover the pot and cook until the beans are fully cooked. Season with salt and let sit 20 minutes. Retaste for seasoning, adjust as necessary, and serve.

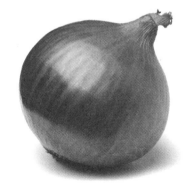

SOUTHERN-STYLE GREEN BEAN SOUP

SERVES 4–6

I love traveling through the South, stopping at buffets and barbeque joints. At any of these places along the way, you'll find a tray of green beans simmering away—the inspiration for this dish. The green beans cook down to a delightful texture, and the other vegetables provide a rich pairing with the beans. It's a dish that keeps warm well, making it a great choice for entertaining. However, if it is chilled immediately after preparation and reheated the next day, you will find it at its peak.

6   *cups water*

½   *ounce dried kombu*

1   *bay leaf*

3   *tablespoons extra virgin olive oil*

1   *onion, diced*

2   *stalks celery, sliced*

1   *bulb fennel, diced*

2   *garlic cloves, sliced*

2   *pounds green beans, cut into ½-inch pieces*

½   *lemon*

1   *tablespoon vinegar, plus more as needed*
    Salt
    Vinegar-based hot sauce

1. In a large pot, combine the water, kombu, bay leaf, olive oil, onion, celery, fennel, and garlic and bring to a simmer. Cook for 45 minutes.

2. Remove the kombu, cut it into small pieces, and return it to the pot. Discard the bay leaf.

3. Add the green beans, lemon half, and vinegar, and season with salt. Simmer for 20 minutes.

4. Remove from the heat. Squeeze the lemon and discard the peel. Adjust seasoning with salt and vinegar if necessary.

5. Serve with a good dash of vinegar-based hot sauce.

ARSENIC

Arsenic is an element that naturally exists in the air, soil, and water in which our food is grown. Organic and inorganic forms of arsenic are present in many foods, such as fruits, vegetables, grains, and seafood, as well as water, wine, and juices, among others. The FDA regulates the levels of arsenic in all food products, so you need not worry about arsenic consumption. In addition, the Food Safety Modernization Act of 2011 ensures that foods imported into the United States are safe for consumers. Eating seagreens purchased from regulated businesses is no riskier than consuming any other produce.

SEAGREEN VEGETABLE SOUP

SERVES 4–6

In this dish, the light flavor of chicken broth is paired with the anise/licorice aroma of fennel and the meaty flavor of bok choy, another superfood. This soup is easy to make if you have broth on hand. So, with a little planning, a quick lunch or dinner can be made by pulling a quart or two of stock out of the freezer, adding the vegetables, and simmering.

1 *bulb fennel, diced*

1 *large bok choy, chopped*

3 *celery stalks, sliced*

1 *tablespoon lemon juice*

1 *stalk lemongrass, beaten**

¾ *ounce dried kombu, flaked into ½-inch pieces*

6 *cups Chicken and Seagreen Stock (see page 113)*

   Salt

3 *scallions, cut into 1-inch segments*

½ *bunch basil, leaves only*

1 *serrano chile, sliced thin*

1. Add the fennel, bok choy, celery, lemon juice, lemongrass, kombu, and stock to a large pot. Season with salt and simmer until the vegetables are tender.

2. Remove the lemongrass.

3. Garnish with scallions, basil, and slices of serrano chile.

*Simply bruise the whole stalk of lemongrass, using a metal spoon or the blunt side of a knife, to release oils and aroma.

FIERY-HOT BUTTER BEAN AND ESCAROLE SOUP

SERVES 4–6

It's up to you to decide how fiery hot you want this soup to be. I tend to add even more heat than the recipe calls for and let the smoothness of the butter beans and cool green escarole soften the blow.

8 *tablespoons extra virgin olive oil*

1 *bulb fennel, diced*

1 *onion, diced*

6 *cloves garlic, crushed*

1 *ounce dulse flakes*

1–2 *tablespoons chile flakes*

1 *head escarole, chopped into bite-size pieces*

2 *(15 ounce) cans butter beans, drained and rinsed*

1½ *quarts seagreen stock (see pages 111–113)*

   Salt

4 *tablespoons grated Parmesan cheese*

1 *baguette*

1. In 4 tablespoons of the olive oil, sauté the fennel, onion, and garlic until they turn translucent, about 5 minutes.

2. Add the dulse and chile flakes, and toss to combine.

3. Add the escarole, butter beans, and stock. Season with salt. Simmer for 20 minutes over low heat.

4. Remove from the heat and allow to rest 5 minutes.

5. Garnish with Parmesan, and drizzle with the remaining olive oil. Serve with a warm baguette.

PHO WITH SHRIMP

SERVES 4–6

This take on a traditional, heartwarming Vietnamese soup can use almost any form of seafood. I like shrimp in particular because it's a crowd pleaser, the shells add so much depth and richness to the broth, and it brings the seagreens an added dimension and complexity.

6 *cups seagreen stock (see pages 111–113)*

1 *1-inch knob of fresh ginger, peeled and sliced*

   Pinch celery seed

8 *whole cloves*

4 *bay leaves*

4 *allspice berries*

1 *tablespoon coriander seeds*

1 *pound shrimp in shells*

   Salt

2 *(4 ounce) packages thin pho rice noodles (may substitute vermicelli or angel hair pasta)*

8 *sprigs mint leaves, torn*

½ *red serrano chile, cut into thin rounds*

4 *lime wedges*

1 *cup dried wakame strips*

1. Combine the stock, ginger, celery seed, cloves, bay leaves, allspice, coriander, and shrimp along with a couple healthy pinches of salt, and simmer until the shrimp is just cooked.

2. Peel and set aside the shrimp, add the shells back to the broth, and let steep 10 minutes.

3. Strain the broth, reserve the liquid, and discard the solids.

4. Prepare the noodles in the broth according to the package directions.

5. To serve, divide the noodles among four bowls. Add the shrimp on top. Pour the broth over the noodles and garnish with mint leaves, chile, a lime wedge, and wakame strips.

MISO SOUP

MAKES 2 QUARTS

Many Americans are familiar with this soup, as it is a traditional appetizer in sushi restaurants the country over. With its warming and hearty flavors of fermented miso, rich umami flavor, and gentle nuanced broth, this soup is simple to prepare in just a few minutes. The recipe below makes a wonderful base on which to build your own creations—just add tofu, fresh herbs, chicken, seafood, or whatever you like.

2   quarts Basic Dashi Broth (see page 111)

½   cup red miso paste

1. Combine and bring to a simmer.

2. Optional garnishes: enoki mushrooms, scallions, diced tofu.

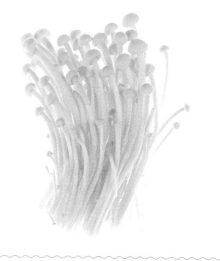

2   quarts Basic Dashi Broth (see page 111)

TRY THESE SPECIAL INGREDIENTS

MISO

Miso is a thick paste of fermented soybean and salt. A traditional Japanese food, it is very high in sodium and is used for marinating other proteins. There are several varieties of miso. Generally, white, yellow, and red varieties are distinguished by the length of time they've been fermented and the amount of salt used. The longer the fermentation, the richer, deeper, and more robust the flavor. Different varieties of miso are used for various purposes. Red miso is the preferred type for the eponymous miso soup.

ENOKI MUSHROOMS

These white mushrooms are very long stemmed and very thin, and have a tiny cap. They are wonderful in raw preparations or in soups, where the heat of the broth lightly wilts the mushrooms, giving them them a pasta-like texture. Enoki have a very mild earthy flavor that pairs well with the umami flavors of dashi and miso.

MOORISH STEW

SERVES 4

This stew, inspired by a dish I enjoyed while I was living in Spain, combines chickpeas and potatoes simmered with an aromatic base of garlic and onions, and laced with the heady scent of smoked paprika. As richly flavored as this dish is, the potatoes absorb and balance these ingredients. The chickpeas add a mellow tone and contrasting texture. Traditionally this stew is thick with wilted spinach, which I've substituted here with seagreens. Like many stews, this one tastes even better if it is left to chill overnight and then reheated and served the next day. Topping it off with a fried egg may gild the lily, but it makes for a very satisfying meal.

3   tablespoons olive oil

1½ pounds red skin or russet potatoes (about 3), peeled and diced into ¾-inch cubes

1   onion, chopped

2   cloves garlic, minced

2   teaspoons smoked paprika
    Salt

3   cups fresh or frozen seagreens or 1 ounce dried, rehydrated

1   (15 ounce) can drained and rinsed chickpeas

4   cups Vegetable and Seagreen Broth (see page 113)

1   (16 ounce) can diced tomatoes

4   eggs, fried (optional)

1. In a Dutch oven, heat the oil over moderate heat. Add the potatoes and onion and sauté, stirring frequently, until the potatoes start to brown, about 5 minutes. Add the garlic, paprika, and salt, and cook, stirring, until fragrant, about 1 minute.

2. Add the seagreens, chickpeas, broth, and tomatoes. Bring to a simmer and cook until the potatoes are tender, about 15 minutes. Season with salt and serve. Garnish each bowl with a fried egg, if desired.

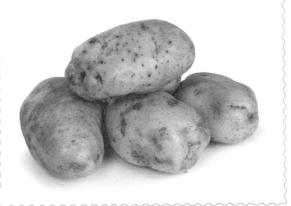

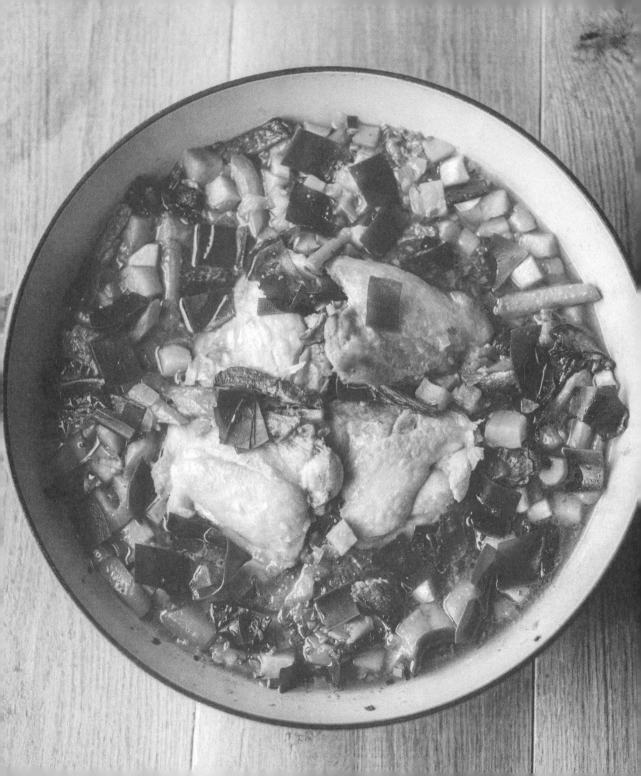

CHAPTER 11

LARGER DISHES

More often than not, given the robust flavor of seagreens, they are integrated into dishes, rather than celebrated outright, on their own. The dishes that follow are an opportunity to put seagreens front and center, whether it be in a family favorite such as lasagna or an interesting and exotic preparation such as the classic Indian dish saag paneer. For many of these recipes, it's best to use fresh or frozen seagreens, while in others, where their application is more appropriate, I recommend using dried seagreens. Given the quantity of seagreens in many of the recipes that follow, you might want to give yourself a gentler introduction to these unique greens by gradually integrating them into your regular weekly menus (see page 52) before diving into a full entrée.

DASHI-BRAISED CHICKEN WITH ROOT VEGETABLES

SERVES 4

This comforting dish of braised chicken and root vegetables is made all the more exciting with the rich umami flavors of the seagreens, although the resulting dish is just as familiar and comforting as something Grandma would make.

- 4 bone-in, skin-on chicken thighs
   Salt
- 5 tablespoons peanut or olive oil
- 1 bunch scallions
- 1 clove garlic, minced
- 1 teaspoon grated fresh ginger
- ½ ounce dried shiitake or porcini mushrooms
- 1 medium yellow onion, sliced
- 2 medium turnips, peeled and cut into 1-inch pieces
- 4 medium Yukon Gold potatoes, peeled and cut into 1-inch pieces
- 2 carrots, cut into 1-inch pieces
- 2 cups Basic Dashi Broth (see page 111)
- 2 tablespoons rice wine vinegar
- ¼ cup soy sauce
- ½ cup chopped seagreens (reserved from broth, or add ¼ cup dried kelp flakes)

1. Season the chicken with salt.

(continued)

2. Heat 1 tablespoon of the oil in a large cast-iron pan and sear the chicken until golden brown. Remove the chicken from the pan and set aside.

3. In the remaining oil, cook the scallions, garlic, and ginger. Add the mushrooms and onion, and cook until just wilted. Add the turnips, potatoes, and carrots, and toss to combine. Nestle the chicken legs among the vegetables.

4. Add the broth, vinegar, soy sauce, and seagreens. Cover and bring to a simmer. Cook on low heat until the chicken is cooked through, about 25 minutes.

5. Divide the chicken between four shallow bowls and ladle the vegetables and broth over top.

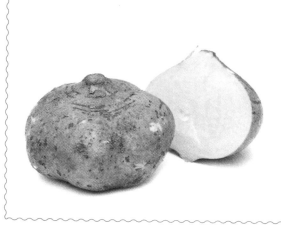

SAAG PANEER

SERVES 6

This classic vegetarian Indian dish is easy to whip up in large batches, making it ideal to serve with meals throughout the week. In this version of the dish, spinach is paired with kombu—a powerful nutritional combo—and it's a great way to introduce your family to seagreens through a more familiar dish. Paneer (Indian cheese) is available at specialty grocery stores and easy to make at home. You can also substitute Halloumi cheese or tofu.

9   *ounces paneer or Halloumi cheese, cut into 1-inch cubes*

2   *tablespoons butter*

1   *onion, sliced fine*

4   *cloves garlic*

1   *hot pepper, minced*

1   *teaspoon ground ginger*

1   *teaspoon ground cumin*

1 *teaspoon ground coriander*

1   *(10 ounce) package frozen spinach*

½   *ounce dried kombu, rehydrated in 1 cup water*

   Salt

1   *cup Basic Dashi Broth (see page 111)*

½   *cup plain yogurt (not Greek yogurt)*

1. Sear the paneer in the butter; set aside. In the same pan, sauté the onion, garlic, hot pepper, ginger, cumin, and coriander. Add the spinach and kombu and stir well. Season with salt and add the dashi. Cook about 5 minutes.

2. Turn the heat off. Add the yogurt, a little at a time to keep it from curdling. Once the yogurt is well mixed into the greens, add the paneer. Turn the heat back on, cover, and cook until everything is warmed through, about 5 minutes. Serve.

STIR-FRIED SEAGREENS

SERVES 4–6

Stir-frying is a method more than a strict recipe. Here, a combination of the superfoods bok choy, carrots, and seagreens brings great flavor, texture, and color to the mix. Peanuts add crunch and a protein boost. The stir-fry technique can be used with any mixture of ingredients. The key is to start with an aromatic flavor base of ginger, garlic, and scallion, cooked over extremely high heat in a pan that holds heat well in order to avoid steaming the ingredients.

¼ cup peanut oil

1 tablespoon grated fresh ginger

4 cloves garlic, sliced

1 bunch scallions, finely sliced

1 cup peanuts, crushed

1 pound bok choy or napa cabbage, sliced

3 carrots, grated

2 ounces dried kombu, rehydrated and sliced

¼ cup oyster sauce or hoisin sauce

2 tablespoons soy sauce

2 tablespoons rice wine vinegar
   Salt

1. In a large, heavy-bottomed pan, heat the oil over high heat. Add the ginger, garlic, scallions, and peanuts, and cook for just a few seconds in the hot oil. Add the bok choy or cabbage and carrots and toss to thoroughly coat with hot oil; let sit until the bok choy begins to wilt and slightly color. Add the seagreens. Toss to combine and cook until heated through.

2. In a separate bowl, whisk together the oyster sauce or hoisin sauce, soy sauce, and rice wine vinegar, then add to the cooking vegetables. Toss to combine.

3. Season with salt and serve. This is great with Umami-Rich Rice Pilaf (see page 94).

DID YOU KNOW?

Ancient Roman records indicate that seaweeds were used to treat skin wounds, burns, and rashes.

LASAGNA

SERVES 6–8

What's more comforting than lasagna? It's easy to make ahead of time and better when done so. It's easy to reheat and provides leftovers the week through. Hey, it's lasagna. Everyone loves it.

- 1 *pound lasagna noodles*
- 3 *tablespoons olive oil*
- 1 *clove garlic, minced*
- 1 *onion, diced*
- 4 *tablespoons dulse flakes*
- 1 *pound 95 percent lean ground beef, chicken, or turkey*
-    *Salt*

- 1 *(28 ounce) can crushed tomatoes*
- ½ *tablespoon dried oregano*
- 1 *teaspoon chile flakes*
- 15 *ounces ricotta cheese*
- 1 *ounce dried kelp, rehydrated, then cut into strips*

1. Boil the noodles according to the instructions on the package. Drain and set aside.

2. Preheat the oven to 325°F. In the oil, cook the garlic, onion, and dulse until aromatic, about 2 minutes. Add the beef and cook until it begins to brown and is nearly cooked through. Season with salt and add the tomatoes, oregano, and chile flakes. Bring to a simmer, then remove from the heat.

WINE WITH SEAGREENS

Given the unique flavors of seagreens, pairing them with wine might seem a bit daunting. In fact, the heavy umami flavors lent to food by seagreens can really kick the flavors of red wines into overdrive. In particular, I've found that dulse can amazingly flatter a robust and fruity California cabernet. The more delicately flavored wakame and kelp do wonders for lighter, fruitier reds such as pinot noir, Beaujolais, and cabernet franc. White wines are certainly on the menu as well. The heavier, more distinct styles pair best. Gewürztraminer, Viognier, pinot gris, and the lighter but ebulliently flavored Riesling are well adapted to dishes flavored lightly with seagreens, especially soups. For dishes that contain a significant amount of seagreens, such as Sauteed Seagreens with Bacon, Apple, and Onion (page 91), the pairing can be a little more difficult, as the flavors of the seagreens, though not overwhelming to the palate, can overwhelm the wine just due to volume of flavor. When pairing wines, there is no such thing as a wrong choice. If you like the wine and you like the food, then who's to tell you otherwise?

3. In a baking dish, layer the ingredients in this order: half of the noodles, half of the beef, half of the cheese, all of the kelp, the remaining noodles, the remaining beef, and the remaining cheese.

4. Bake until the lasagna is bubbling and the cheese is lightly browned, about 45 minutes.

ZUCCHINI AND SEAGREENS "SPAGHETTI" WITH GARLIC

SERVES 4

Making noodles from zucchini is a fun and interesting way to add more vegetables to a meal while satisfying our cravings for the familiar pleasures of pasta. In this case, the zucchini serves in place of the noodle. It cooks very quickly, and its texture is complemented by the slight crunch of the seagreens.

2   *ounces dried kelp, rehydrated; reserve ½ cup of liquid*

6   *large zucchini (about 3 pounds)*

3   *tablespoons butter*

3   *cloves garlic, sliced thin*

1   *cup parsley, leaves only*

   Salt

   Freshly cracked pepper

1. Chop the kelp into ribbons about the thickness of linguini.

2. Either by hand or using a mandoline, finely julienne the zucchini, rotating around the outside, leaving behind the inner seeded flesh.

3. Heat the butter and garlic over medium heat in a covered pan for 3 minutes. Add the zucchini, kelp, and 3 tablespoons of the reserved rehydrating water. Continue to cook over medium heat, approximately 3 minutes. The zucchini will release its juices, combining with the kelp broth and butter to form a nice sauce.

4. When the zucchini has wilted, add the parsley and salt and toss to combine. Check the seasoning and adjust if necessary. Give it a few turns of freshly cracked pepper just prior to serving.

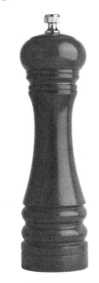

ORECCHIETTE WITH SAUSAGE, SWEET POTATOES, AND SEAGREENS

SERVES 4–6

Orecchiette are ear-shaped pasta that hold sauce very well and pair beautifully with savory ingredients such as sausage and almost any combination of vegetables, herbs, beans, and legumes. This is a dish that my wife and I make at least once a month, and the leftovers, which are delicious eaten cold, provide at least a couple more meals.

- 1 *pound orecchiette pasta*
- 2 *ounces dried kelp, crumbled*
- 1 *pound spicy Italian sausage, removed from its casing*
- 1 *pound sweet potatoes, peeled and diced small*
- 2 *tablespoons olive oil*

1. Bring a pot of salted water to a boil and add the orecchiette and kelp. Cook according to the pasta package instructions until al dente. Strain and reserve 1 cup of cooking liquid.

2. At the same time, in a large pot, sauté the sausage and sweet potatoes in the olive oil, breaking up the sausage into small pieces as it cooks.

3. Once the sausage is cooked, add the pasta and seagreens and the reserved cooking liquid. Bring to a boil and cook until the sauce is thickened and the sweet potatoes are fully cooked, 3–4 minutes.

SEAGREEN-WRAPPED ROASTED ROOT VEGETABLES

Rehydrating sheets of seagreens such as kombu or dulse provides an excellent way to add flavor and nutrition to root vegetables. The technique is the same for just about anything—potatoes, sweet turnips, carrots, you name it. With the tip of the paring knife, pierce the root vegetable all over, rub with olive oil, and season with salt. Lay out a piece of parchment paper. Cover with a layer of seagreens large enough to wrap all around the vegetable. Place the vegetable in the center and wrap the parchment around the vegetable. Place on a baking sheet with the folded edge underneath, so as to keep the package closed. Roast at 350°F for about 40 minutes. Cut open the parchment tableside to release the delicious aromas and serve with salt, pepper, and olive oil as accompaniments, if you like.

SEAFOOD OR CHICKEN CHILI VERDE

SERVES 4

Chili verde is a wonderfully hearty dish with all of the fiery character of Tex-Mex cooking, but with a fresh and vibrant set of flavors not often associated with the richness of that cuisine. Chili verde is a combination of fresh herbs and seagreens puréed with tomatillos to form a zippy base for the soup, rich with potatoes and chicken, swordfish, or pork, simmered into a chunky and satisfying meal.

¼ *cup olive oil*

1 *large yellow onion, roughly chopped*

1 *bulb fennel, roughly chopped*

2 *Anaheim or poblano chiles (or other medium-hot pepper of your choice, or spicier if you want)*

5 *cloves garlic, peeled and sliced*

1 *tablespoon dried oregano*

1 *ounce dried kelp*

½ *pound tomatillos, husks removed and washed well, cut into quarters*

4 *cups water*

1 *bunch cilantro*

1 *bunch scallions*

   Salt

1½ *pounds seafood, such as swordfish or a large, flaked whitefish such as Pacific cod or rockfish, or 1½ pounds chicken thighs*

1. In a large sauté pan, heat the oil over high heat and cook the onion and fennel for approximately 5 minutes until they begin to wilt.

2. Add the chiles, garlic, oregano, and kelp, and cook another 5 minutes.

3. Add the tomatillos and water. Bring to a simmer and cook until the tomatillos are completely soft and falling apart.

4. Transfer the mixture to a high-speed blender such as a Vitamix and blend to a smooth purée. Once puréed, add the cilantro and scallions and purée until smooth.

5. Add the purée back to the pan and adjust the seasoning with salt as necessary.

6. Add the seafood or chicken to the purée and simmer over low heat until fully cooked; the cooking time depends on which protein you are using.

7. When cooked, let rest for 20 minutes off the heat, then serve over Umami-Rich Rice Pilaf (see page 94).

VEGGIE BURGER

MAKES 4 LARGE BURGERS

Seagreen powder enlivens veggie burgers just as magically as it transforms traditional beef burgers, adding a rich umami layer and bringing all of the nutritious ingredients into delicious balance.

- 2   *tablespoons extra virgin olive oil*
- 1   *shallot or small onion, minced*
- 1   *clove garlic, grated on a Microplane grater or very finely minced*
- 2   *tablespoons chopped walnuts*
- 1   *tablespoon smoked sweet paprika*
- 4   *pitted prunes, roughly chopped*
- 1   *medium beet, boiled in water to cover until tender, peeled, and shredded on the large holes of a box grater*
- 2   *tablespoons red wine vinegar*
- 2   *cups cooked brown rice (follow instructions on the package)*
- 1   *(15 ounce) can black beans, drained and briefly rinsed*
- 5   *tablespoons oat bran or instant oatmeal*
- 3   *tablespoons powdered kelp*
- 1   *large egg (optional)*
     Kosher Salt

1. Heat 1½ tablespoons of the olive oil in a small skillet over medium heat and cook the shallot and garlic until translucent, about 5 minutes. Add the walnuts and paprika, toss to combine, and cook 1 minute more. Add the prunes, shredded beet, and vinegar. Stir to combine and remove from the heat.

2. In a large bowl, combine the beet mixture with the rice, beans, oat bran, kelp, and egg, if using. Season generously with salt. Stir with some force to mash most of the beans and rice into a tacky paste that still has some chunks. Taste for seasoning and adjust if necessary. Chill the mixture for at least an hour.

3. Form the chilled mixture into four patties, each about 1 inch thick. Brush them with the remaining olive oil, then sear in a pan, under the broiler, or over a grill. When they begin to crisp and brown, carefully flip the patties over and cook for another few minutes to heat through, about 5 minutes.

USING SEAGREENS TO WRAP FISH OR CHICKEN FOR THE GRILL

Fresh seagreens in nearly any form, from rockweed to kelp, can be used to wrap whole fish, fillets, or chicken prior to baking or grilling. If need be, you can use twine to lightly bind the wrapping. This will not only help prevent the seafood from sticking to the grill but will also imbue the flesh with the perfume of sea-salty air.

UMAMI-SPIKED BURGER

MAKES 4 BURGERS

You'll be amazed at what the addition of seagreens does for the flavor of ground beef. The richness and depth of flavor is so surprising that you will certainly have people asking you what your secret is.

2 teaspoons onion powder

2 teaspoons garlic powder

3 tablespoons dulse flakes (applewood-smoked is preferable) or 1 tablespoon kelp powder

  Fresh cracked pepper

1 teaspoon ground allspice

  Salt

1¼ pound ground beef

1. Mix all the ingredients together. Form patties and grill to desired doneness.

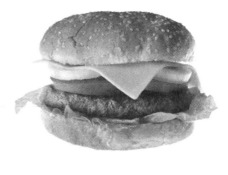

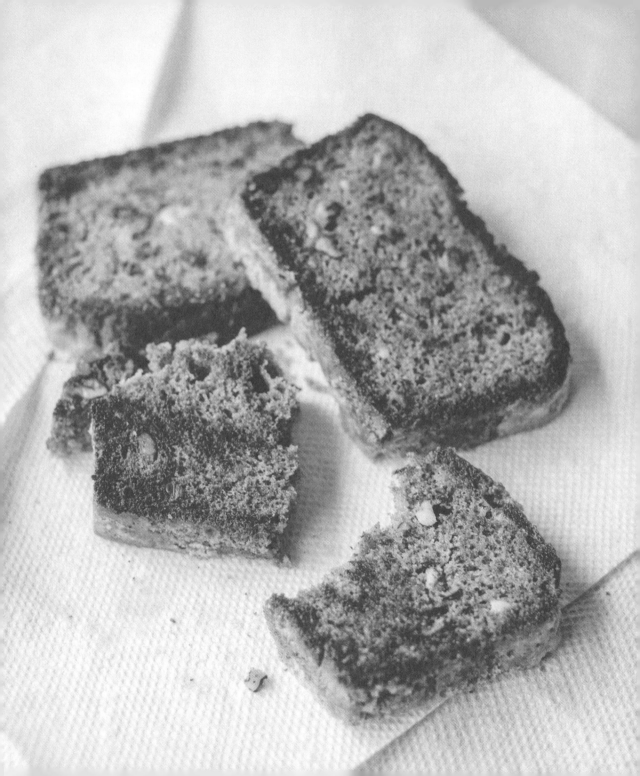

CHAPTER 12

BREADS, MUFFINS, AND DESSERTS

Baked goods and desserts are ideal for hiding seagreens, should someone be opposed to them—say, a picky child. Given that baked dishes are sweet far more often than not, we tend not to think of savory flavors as the predominant characteristic, and in the recipes that follow this holds true. Seagreens, usually in a dried form, can easily substitute for some of an ingredient like flour, adding flavor and nutrition but not necessarily taking its place in terms of recipe dynamics. In a recipe for cake, the flavor of seagreens melts away into a rich, velvety, chocolaty flavor. And seagreens stand shoulder-to-shoulder with zucchini as ideal ingredients in all kinds of delicious breads, muffins, and desserts. Baking with seagreens is an adventure. Be bold. The next time you make banana bread, add a tablespoon or two of seagreens—and watch what happens. People won't stop asking you for the mystery ingredient.

SEEDED MULTIGRAIN BREAD

MAKES 1 LOAF

Put as many or as few seagreens into this bread as you care to. I particularly like dulse flakes, as the dark purple flecks add a nice visual punctuation to the bread. It is especially good when sliced and toasted and then slathered with almond or peanut butter.

- 1¼ cups whole wheat flour
- 1 cup all-purpose flour
- 2 tablespoons kelp or dulse, powder or flakes
- ½ teaspoon salt
- 3 tablespoons sunflower seeds
- 3 tablespoons sesame seeds
- 3 tablespoons shelled pumpkin seeds
- ⅓ cup rolled oats
- 1 cup water, Basic Dashi Broth (see page 111), or reserved seagreen rehydration water
- 2 tablespoons molasses
- 1 (¼ ounce) package active dry yeast
- 1 egg
- 1 egg white

1. In a large bowl, combine the whole wheat flour, all-purpose flour, seagreens, and salt.

(continued)

OPPOSITE: **Seeded Multigrain Bread, above**

2. In another bowl, mix the sunflower seeds, sesame seeds, pumpkin seeds, and oats, and set aside.

3. In a saucepan, combine the liquid and molasses and warm the mixture over low heat until just it reaches 120°F. Add the yeast and let it bloom. Whisk in the egg. Add the liquid to the flour mixture. Mix together until a soft dough forms.

4. Turn the dough onto a lightly floured surface. Knead for 10 minutes, then shape into a ball.

5. Lightly oil a large stainless steel bowl. Add the dough and turn it to cover the dough with the oil. Cover the bowl with a towel and let rise in a warm place for 2 hours until doubled in size.

6. When the dough has risen, punch the dough down with your fists and add all but 2 tablespoons of the seed mixture, working it into the dough. Shape the dough into a loaf by rolling it into a 12 × 8 inch rectangle, and then roll it up by its shortest end. Pinch the ends together and tuck underneath.

7. Place in a nonstick 9 × 5 inch loaf pan with the seam underneath. Cover the loaf pan with a towel and let rise for 1 hour until doubled in bulk.

8. Preheat the oven to 350°F. Brush the top of the loaf with egg white and sprinkle with the remaining 2 tablespoons of seed mixture. Bake the bread for 30 minutes or until the loaf sounds hollow when tapped on the bottom. Remove the bread from the pan and let it cool completely.

MORNING GLORY MUFFINS
MAKES 12 MUFFINS

A big batch of these muffins made on Sunday morning will last you through the week (maybe—they're pretty good). They're also a great way to use a familiar vehicle to introduce a delicious and nutritious new ingredient into your diet.

1½ cups all-purpose flour

½ cup whole wheat flour

1¼ cups white sugar

2 tablespoons ground cinnamon

1 tablespoon ground ginger

2 teaspoons baking powder

½ teaspoon baking soda

½ teaspoon salt

2 eggs

½ cup puréed fresh seagreens, or ½ cup applesauce with 2 tablespoons flaked or powdered seagreens mixed in

¼ cup vegetable oil

1 tablespoon vanilla extract

2 cups grated carrots

1 apple, peeled, cored, and chopped

1 cup raisins

2 tablespoons chopped walnuts

1. Preheat the oven to 375°F. Grease or line a muffin tin.

2. In a bowl, whisk together the all-purpose flour, whole wheat flour, sugar, cinnamon, ginger, baking powder, baking soda, and salt.

3. In another bowl, combine the eggs, seagreens, oil, and vanilla extract.

4. Add the wet ingredients to the dry ingredients. Stir in carrots, apple, raisins, and walnuts and mix until all ingredients are just combined.

5. Spoon the batter into the greased or lined muffin tin, filling them about three-quarters full.

6. Bake for 15–20 minutes or until the tops are golden and spring back when lightly pressed.

ZUCCHINI-SEAGREEN BREAD

MAKES 2 LOAVES

In making this recipe, I was so surprised by how seamlessly the seagreens integrated with the personality of the bread. You can easily replace the zucchini altogether by doubling the seagreens with delicious results.

3 cups all-purpose flour

1 teaspoon salt

1 teaspoon baking soda

1 teaspoon baking powder

1 tablespoon ground cinnamon

3 eggs

1 cup vegetable oil

3 teaspoons vanilla extract

2¼ cups white sugar

1 cup grated zucchini

10 sheets nori, chopped and rehydrated in ½ cup water

1 cup chopped walnuts

1. Grease and flour two 8 × 4 inch loaf pans. Preheat the oven to 325°F.

2. Sift the flour, salt, baking soda, baking powder, and cinnamon together in a bowl.

3. In a separate large bowl, beat the eggs, oil, vanilla, and sugar together.

(continued)

4. Add the sifted ingredients to the creamed mixture, and beat well. Stir in the zucchini, seagreens, and nuts until well combined.

5. Pour the batter into the prepared pans. Bake for 40–60 minutes, or until a tester inserted in the center comes out clean.

6. Cool in pan on a rack for 20 minutes. Remove the bread from pan, and cool completely.

CHOCOLATE CAKE

MAKES ONE 9 × 13 INCH CAKE

Hey, it's chocolate cake. Who cares if it has seagreens in it. Even the most finicky eater will dive into this one. And anyone seeking nutritive benefits won't feel so much as a twinge of sacrifice when enjoying this dish.

2½ cups all-purpose flour

2½ teaspoons baking powder

1½ teaspoons baking soda

1 teaspoon salt

1 teaspoon ground cinnamon

½ cup unsweetened cocoa powder

8 tablespoons (1 stick) unsalted butter, softened

¼ cup vegetable oil

2 cups white sugar

3 eggs

1 teaspoon vanilla extract

2 cups finely minced seagreens, fresh, frozen, or rehydrated

1. Preheat the oven to 350°F. Grease and flour a 9 × 13 inch pan.

2. Sift together the flour, baking powder, baking soda, salt, cinnamon, and cocoa powder. Set aside.

3. In a large bowl, cream together the butter, oil, and sugar until light and fluffy. Beat in the eggs, one at a time, then stir in the vanilla and seagreens. Mix the liquid ingredients into the dry ingredients, and mix until just combined.

4. Pour the batter into the prepared pan. Bake for 55–60 minutes, or until a toothpick inserted into the center of the cake comes out clean. Allow to cool.

BLANCMANGE

SERVES 4

You wouldn't think that seagreens would find a place in any dessert, but their thickening properties have long been used in the form of agar, as a cheap and easy substitute for eggs in custard preparations. This recipe for blancmange can be used as a base for flavored puddings with chocolate or nuts, for example, simply by adding those ingredients once the agar has dissolved in the warm milk.

- 2 cups milk
- 1 tablespoon agar flakes (a seaweed-based gelatin found at health food stores) or powdered gelatin
- ¼ cup honey
- 1 vanilla bean, cut lengthwise and seeds scraped, or 2 teaspoons vanilla extract

  Lemon zest

  Cinnamon

1. Pour the milk into a medium saucepan and sprinkle the agar on top. Allow to rest until the agar becomes clear and puffs slightly, 10–15 minutes.

2. Bring the milk to a simmer and cook, stirring often, until the flakes dissolve, 1–2 minutes. Add the honey, vanilla seeds, lemon zest to taste, and cinnamon to taste. Chill and let set for 2 hours.

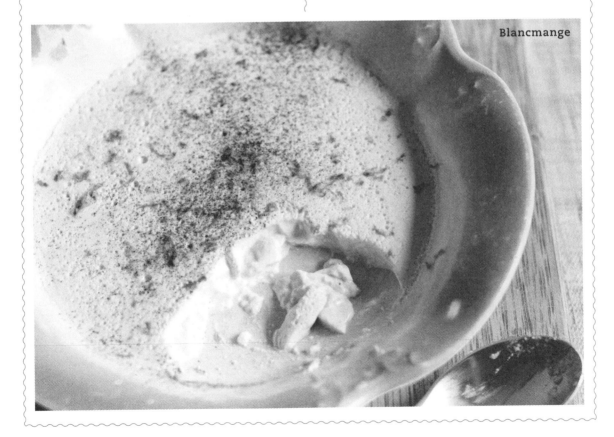

Blancmange

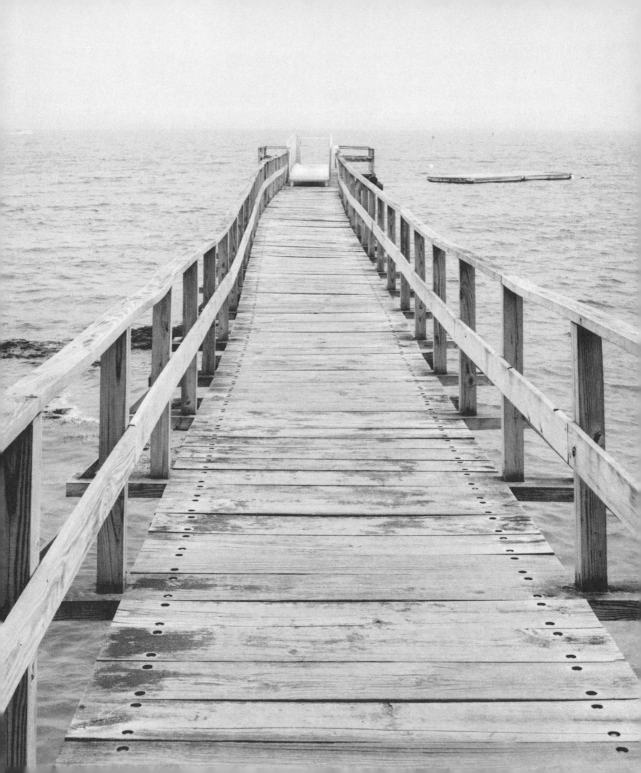

CHAPTER 13

FREQUENTLY ASKED QUESTIONS

When learning about a new ingredient such as seagreens—and all of its incredible benefits—there's bound to be questions and misconceptions. Here are some of the questions I am most frequently asked regarding this incredible ingredient.

BASIC INFORMATION

What are seagreens?

Seagreens are water-based algae that can be harvested in the wild or cultivated as aquaculture, but we treat them like vegetables and leafy greens.

Why are there so many names and terms for seagreens?

The terminology used for seagreens is indeed vast. Seagreens are referred to by their scientific as well as their regional and colloquial names. I use *seagreens* as a broad term for all edible seaweeds. Other generic names are algae, macroalgae, marine plants, sea vegetables, and so on. Species are divided into green, red, and brown seagreens, and they have common names such as kelp, nori, alaria, wakame, sea lettuce, and so on. Don't get put off by these names; experiment with the forms you can find and enjoy them in wide variety of recipes, such as the ones in this book.

Are all seaweeds edible?

The majority of seaweeds are edible, but I tend to err on the side of caution and stick with the ones that are commercially available. Some wild-harvested seagreens can be quite unpalatable or may have high levels of toxins, depending on where they are grown.

Are seagreens good for me?

In short, yes! They are rich in minerals, vitamins, and fiber among other nutritious elements.

Do seagreens taste "fishy"?

Not at all. They can have a briny salinity or an umami savoriness, but they definitely do not taste fishy. Some seagreens have a slight seawater flavor, and because they are so nutrient dense, a little goes a long way.

How are seagreens dried?

There are different processes for drying seagreens—sun drying, low temperature air-drying, and traditional dehydrator drying are some of the methods. Most producers will list this on their packaging or website.

NUTRIENTS

What vitamins, minerals, and nutrients are found in seagreens?

Seagreens can contain more than fifty vitamins and minerals, including vitamin A, C, vitamin B_6, vitamin B_{12}, folate, vitamin D, calcium, potassium, magnesium, phosphorus, iron, protein, iodine, sulfur, sodium alginate, and sterols.

What's the difference between a vitamin and a mineral?

Vitamins are organic substances created by plants or animals, whereas minerals are inorganic elements that are absorbed by plants from soil and water.

Can seagreens help me lose weight?

There is no magic food that will help you shed unwanted pounds. A healthy diet full of a diversity of plant-based foods and lean proteins are certainly essential to any weight-loss program. That said, seagreens can greatly augment a healthy diet as they are low in calories, nutrient dense, and very low in unsaturated fat (less than 2 percent). The iodine in seagreens can stimulate the thyroid to speed metabolism, and fiber helps to both stimulate the digestive tract and increase feelings of fullness.

What is the difference between soluble and insoluble fiber?

Soluble fiber dissolves in water and forms a gel-like substance that may help lower blood glucose and cholesterol levels. It can be found in oats, peas, beans, apples, and citrus fruits. Insoluble fiber does not dissolve in water and passes through the digestive tract, providing stool bulk. It can be found in whole grains, nuts, legumes, and many vegetables. Seagreens have both soluble and insoluble fiber.

How much fiber do seagreens have?

Dulse, kelp, alaria, and nori are approximately 30 percent total fiber, about equal portions soluble and insoluble.

How much iron is in seagreens?

About ⅓ cup (¼ ounce) serving of dulse or kelp gives up to 30 percent of the RDA of iron, four times the iron in spinach.

How much calcium is in seagreens?

A ½-cup serving of alaria contains more calcium than ½ cup boiled kale or bok choy.

How much magnesium is in seagreens?

Magnesium is twice as abundant in kelp and alaria than in collard greens and exceeds the amount in walnuts, bananas, potatoes, oatmeal, and even sockeye salmon.

How much protein do seagreens have?

Depending on size and growing conditions of the seagreen, protein content can be up to 25 percent by weight. Red seagreens (dulse and laver) generally have more protein than brown seagreens (kelp and alaria).

SEAGREENS AND HEALTH

Can seagreens interfere with blood-thinning medications?

Seagreens do contain vitamin K, so it is important to check with your health-care provider before adding them to your diet if you are on blood-thinning medications. However, when seagreens are consumed in normal quantities, the vitamin K content should not be high enough to cause harmful interactions.

I have high blood pressure and have to limit my salt intake. Can I eat seagreens?

Sodium is an essential mineral. In our modern diet it is often used in excess. Naturally occurring sodium in seagreens is balanced by potassium, magnesium, and calcium, making it ideal for consumption. Because of this balanced saltiness, it may even be a good flavoring alternative for other foods. As with any new food, always consult your health-care practitioner about your individual needs.

I've heard seagreens can reduce the risk of some cancers. Is this true?

Some medical research supports this hypothesis. The fucoidan in brown algaes may prevent growth of cancer cells. Many scientists hypothesize that the low incidence of benign and malignant breast disease in Japanese women can be attributed to frequent consumption of seagreens.

What other diseases and conditions may be aided by seagreens?

Some studies link seagreen consumption to lowered risk, easing of symptoms, and even potential cures for conditions ranging from hypertension and diabetes to arthritis. Seagreens may also reduce the symptoms of difficult pregnancies. Consult with your medical practitioner for more specific information regarding seagreen consumption and medical conditions.

I've heard seagreens can help in detoxification. How? What does this mean?

Detoxification can mean many things. Heavy metal poisoning is frequently treated with alginic acid, a polysaccharide found in kelp and alaria. It can bind with toxic molecules and reduce absorption of strontium 90 and heavy metals such as cadmium. Seaweed consumption can block absorption in the thyroid gland of radioactive iodine-131, found in the atmosphere (especially related to nuclear reactions).

Is it true that seagreens are anti-inflammatory and antiviral?

Fucoidan, a water-soluble compound found in brown algae, has been shown to have both anti-inflammatory and antiviral properties.

CHOOSING, BUYING, AND STORING SEAGREENS

Where can I buy seagreens?

Once you start looking, you will see dried seagreens readily available almost everywhere, from your local health food store to Whole Foods Market to big-box grocery stores! If you can't find one you're looking for, ask your local store to stock it, or order it online.

What forms do seagreens come in?

You can buy seagreens in a variety of forms: dried (whole, flaked, powdered), seasoning mixes, frozen (in a variety of shapes), and fresh (in select markets).

How should I store unused dried seagreens?

Store unused dry seagreens in an airtight container away from moisture and direct sunlight.

How long can seagreens be stored?

Dried seagreens (including leaves, flakes, and powders) have the longest shelf life. Keep them in a cool, dry place and they can last one to two years. Store dried seagreeens in an airtight container out of direct sunlight. Pay attention to expiration dates on packaging.

Fresh, blanched seagreens last about one week in refrigeration. Frozen seagreens will last four to six months.

If seagreens are exposed to moisture, mold, or deterioration, discard them. Discard any seagreens with visible mold or if a mushroom-like aroma develops.

My seagreens have a white powdery substance on them. Is this mold?

Probably not. As seagreens dry, salts and sugars precipitate on the surface. They are safe to eat and are the principal component of seagreens' umami flavor. (You can rinse them if you like, though this does somewhat diminish their flavor.)

Do seagreens freeze well?

Yes! Freeze seagreens on a sheet tray in a single layer, or blend and freeze them in ice cube trays to add to smoothies, soups, and sauces later.

GROWING SEAGREENS

How fast do seagreens grow?

Kelp can grow faster than tropical bamboo, up to ten to twelve inches per day. Under ideal conditions, giant kelp may grow up to two feet each day.

What types of water are best for seagreen growth?

Seagreens can grow in freshwater and saltwater in a wide variety of climates. The seagreens featured in the recipes in this book are all harvested from saltwater.

Can I harvest or forage for my own seagreens?

You can harvest your own seagreens, depending on your location and the time of year. Contact your local Sea Grant or Department of Natural Resources branch for guidelines and regulations for harvesting seagreens in your area.

How are marine plants different from land-based plants?

Because of their requirements to thrive, marine plants are quite different from land-based plants. Marine plants do not need the same structured root, stem, leaf, or vascular tissue of land-based plants. Instead, seagreens have a holdfast, which is used to anchor them to docks, rocks, coral, or other seaweeds as they grow. While land-based plants get their nutrients from soil, marine plants absorb nutrients and minerals from the water environment.

Marine plants are similar to land-based plants in that both use the process of photosynthesis to transform the energy of sunlight, water, and carbon dioxide into chlorophyll and sugars (energy).

Are seagreens sustainable?

Yes. Seagreens are both harvested from the wild and farmed. With any wild harvest of a resource, it is important that the take be managed to allow the resource to maintain a healthy population as well as provide habitat and ecosystem services for its surrounding environment. Cultivated seagreens are a sustainable crop because they do not damage and deplete the environments in which they are grown. In fact, seagreen farming systems help improve the quality of the ecosystems in which they are produced, as they use more carbon than they create.

Are seagreens hard to grow?

Growing seagreens from seed is labor intensive, but the technology and systems that support their cultivation are constantly improving and changing, making aquaculture-grown seagreens a commercially viable product.

What fertilizers are given to seagreens?

Seagreens require zero additional inputs (no fertilizers) in order to grow; all the nutrients they need are taken from natural sources.

COOKING WITH SEAGREENS

Why do some recipes call for a specific type of seagreens, but others just say seagreens?

The recipes in this book are designed to be flexible in terms of the type of seagreen or seagreen product that can be used. In most cases any variety of seagreen will work. The exception is when making a salad, where the volume of a fresh product is needed and cannot be adequately replaced with a dried form. As you substitute, be aware that dried products are far more intense in flavor than fresh seagreens, and powdered seagreens are even stronger in flavor.

Every time I make seagreen chips, they turn chewy. What am I doing wrong?

There are a couple of possible issues here. First, you may not be baking them long enough. Second, you may be using too much oil. You need just a little to add flavor. Try spinning the seagreens in a salad spinner to evenly distribute the oil and avoid excess before you bake the chips. You can also bake them without using any

additional fat. Third, chewiness might also be the result of baking greens when they haven't been adequately dried. Here's a tip: use a lower oven temperature over a longer cooking time, and try blotting seagreens with a tea towel before drying them to get even more moisture out ahead of time. It will speed up the process.

What are the best ways to add seagreens to my diet?

Follow any of the recipes in this book, or use ones you already know. Add seagreens to soups, salads, sauces, marinades, smoothies, and even baked goods.

Should I rinse my seagreens before using?

This is a matter of personal taste. With all but the largest kelps, with visible surface salt, I use them straight out of the bag. If you're using a fresh product, inspect the plants for tiny shells or other marine life before using. Blanching or simply dipping them in cold water will remove any unwanted tagalongs.

I bought a bag of dried seagreens and it has such a strong aroma. I'm afraid to add it to foods.

Don't worry! All dried and concentrated seagreens have a strong smell. When you add them to foods they impart a gentle, savory flavor. But remember, a little goes a long way. Start with ½ teaspoon of dried seagreen flakes or a small section of dried leaves. Test if it is to your liking, then continue to add more and more until it is to your taste.

I'm on a raw diet. Are seagreens appropriate?

Probably. Most domestic dried seagreens (with the exception of pressed nori sheets) are raw products. Imported seagreens may be processed with high heat prior to or in the drying process. Frozen seagreens are usually blanched. Read the information on the package or website for specific product information.

Can I use frozen seagreens the same way I'd use fresh?

For the most part, fresh and frozen seagreens can be used interchangeably in the recipes in this book.

How do I rehydrate seagreens?

Given that the most commonly available form of seagreens is dried, an important first step for many preparations is to reinvigorate the character, texture, and flavor of the seagreens. This is especially important if you are using seagreens in a raw preparation, such as a salad or marinated dish. Seagreens can be rehydrated in almost any form of liquid, which serves two purposes: it removes any caked salt or other minerals that are deposited on the surface of seagreens during the drying process, giving you greater control over the final seasoning of a dish, and it softens the seagreens, making them more pliable, so that they can absorb additional flavors more easily and meld into dishes.

What is umami?

Umami is a savory flavor that occurs naturally in many foods. It is often referred to as the fifth taste, in addition to salty, sweet, sour, and bitter. Umami is defined by a meaty and woodsy flavor.

I want to get my family to eat seagreens, but they are reluctant to try. What should I do?

Try adding it to family-friendly recipes like smoothies, sneaking it into baked goods, and adding dried seagreens to sauces and soups. Start small. Kids frequently love the dried seagreen snacks you can get commercially in different flavors. As with any new food, you may need to try several different methods several different times. When all else fails, add bacon (see page 91).

SEAGREENS AND SAFETY

I've heard seagreens are high in heavy metals and other toxins. Is this true?

This is a common concern. Knowing where your seagreens come from is important, as they do absorb whatever is in the waters in which they grow. Domestic seagreens are harvested in safe waters and tested for safety, so you need not worry about heavy metal contamination. In fact, seagreens are often used to treat heavy metal poisoning! Another way to avoid any concerns about toxicity is to use younger seagreens that have not had as much time in the water and have been exposed to fewer toxins.

Is too much iodine bad for me?

The human body needs 150–1,100 micrograms of dietary iodine daily for healthy thyroid function. If you have a healthy thyroid, excess iodine will be flushed out of your system. However, some people may be more sensitive to excess iodine (nursing mothers, postmenopausal women, or those with thyroid conditions). Before you make any dietary change—and if you have any questions about the safety of iodine consumption—be sure to consult your health-care provider.

I thought iodine was radioactive. Shouldn't we stay away from it?

No. Quite the opposite. Iodine is a necessary dietary element. It is found in hormones produced by the thyroid gland, which regulates our metabolism. Seagreens are perhaps the best source of dietary iodine. Some people are concerned about radioactive iodine, but as long as you are consuming seagreens from safe sources (see page 46), the iodine found in seagreens is iodine-127, which actually blocks absorption of radioactive and toxic iodine-131.

What is carrageenan and what is it used for?

Carrageenan is found in red algae and is used as a natural stabilizer, binding agent, and emulsifier.

I've read that carrageenan is toxic. Is this true?

There are different types of carrageenan. Food-grade carrageenan is natural and safe, and it is found in many products (see page 2). Degraded carrageenan is different from food-grade carrageenan and is a known carcinogen. The controversy over the safety of carrageenan stems from a basic misunderstanding: the harmful effects of carrageenan in its degraded form have been mistakenly associated with food-grade carrageenan, which is safe.

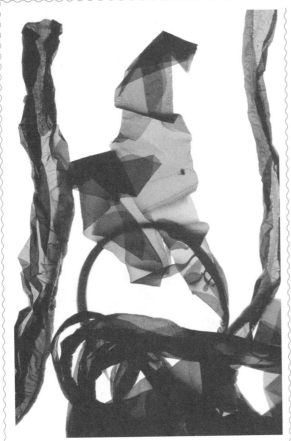

What are potential hazards of seagreen consumption?

Given that seagreens are a product of their environment, they are of course influenced by factors in that environment. Just as vegetables can absorb toxins from the soil, seagreens can absorb them from the water. It's very important that seagreens are harvested where the water quality is tested and safe.

Do seagreens contain arsenic?

Arsenic is an element that naturally exists in the air, soil, and water from which our food is harvested. Organic and inorganic forms of arsenic are present in many foods, such as fruits, vegetables, grains, and seafood, as well as water, wine, and juices, among others. The FDA regulates the level of arsenic in all food ingredients, so you need not worry about arsenic consumption. Furthermore, the Food Safety Modernization Act of 2011 ensures that foods that are imported into the United States are safe for consumers. Seagreens are as safe to buy as any other form of produce from a regulated business.

Is there a risk of contamination by radiation from Fukushima or being irradiated?

Domestically sourced seagreens are tested for safety and are not subject to irradiation, but to ensure your safety and allay any concerns you may have about the safety of seagreens (and anything else you consume, for that matter), find out as much as you can about the product before using it.

NATIONAL INSTITUTE OF HEALTH MEDLINEPLUS

www.nlm.nih.gov/medlineplus

MedlinePlus is the National Institute of Health's website for patients and their families and friends. It is produced by the National Library of Medicine, the world's largest medical library, and features information on diseases, conditions, and wellness issues. It is easy to search and has information for consumers as well as for medical professionals.

MAYO CLINIC HEALTHY LIFESTYLE

www.mayoclinic.org/healthy-lifestyle

Provides easy-to-understand information and tools for a healthy lifestyle.

HARVARD SCHOOL OF PUBLIC HEALTH: DEPARTMENT OF NUTRITION'S NUTRITION SOURCE

www.hsph.harvard.edu/nutritionsource

Provides timely, evidence-based information on diet and nutrition. Information is targeted at both health professionals and the general public. All information is reviewed by a team of professionals, so you can trust its accuracy. As with all websites, it is not intended to offer personal medical advice.

UNIVERSITY OF MARYLAND MEDICAL CENTER COMPLEMENTARY AND ALTERNATIVE MEDICINE GUIDE

umm.edu/health/medical/altmed

This website features information regarding nutrition as a complement to traditional Western medical treatments.

SELF NUTRITION DATA

nutritiondata.self.com

This resource has a number of interactive proprietary tools to analyze and interpret and compare nutritional data.

USDA NATIONAL NUTRIENT DATABASE FOR STANDARD REFERENCE

ndb.nal.usda.gov

Searchable database of nutrient information on more than eight thousand foods.

THE INTERNATIONAL FOOD INFORMATION COUNCIL FOUNDATION

www.foodinsight.org

The International Food Information Council Foundation presents science-based information on health, nutrition, and food safety for the public good. Its searchable database provides information on food safety, among other things.

ACADEMY OF NUTRITION AND DIETETICS EAT RIGHT

www.eatright.org

Articles about topics of interest by members of the Academy of Nutrition and Dietetics. It also provides a search function to put you in touch with a local registered dietitian nutritionist (RDN) in your area to receive personal nutrition counseling.

SUPERKIDS NUTRITION

www.superkidsnutrition.com

Superkids' nutrition website is designed by nutrition experts to provide parents, teachers, dietitians, physicians, nurses, and educators easy to use information for raising healthy kids.

NUTRITION.GOV

www.nutrition.gov

The USDA funded Nutrition.gov features practical information on healthy eating, dietary supplements, fitness and how to keep food safe, containing more than 1000 links to current and reliable nutrition information.

AMERICAN HEART ASSOCIATION NUTRITION CENTER

www.heart.org/HEARTORG

The American Heart Associations put together information on healthy eating, diet and lifestyle recommendations, as well as providing recipes and information about how to buy healthy food in the grocery store and in restaurants.

MAINE SEAWEED FESTIVAL

www.seaweedfest.com

A great event held in my adopted state, the Maine Seaweed Festival sheds light on the use and benefits of seaweed while celebrating the people behind the products. The website also has a host of information on seaweeds.

THIMBLE ISLAND OYSTERS

www.thimbleislandoysters.com/seaweed

More information on Bren Smith, GreenWave, Thimble Island, and three-dimensional farming. (See page 7.)

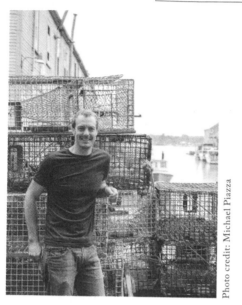

Photo credit: Michael Piazza

BARTON SEAVER, the author of *For Cod & Country* and *Where There's Smoke* (both Sterling Epicure), is quickly establishing himself as the preeminent expert in sustainable seafood. Before leaving the restaurant industry to pursue his interests in sustainable food systems, he created three top restaurants in Washington, DC, and was named Chef of the Year by *Esquire Magazine* in 2009. Seaver's Washington, DC-based restaurant, Hook, was named by *Bon Appétit* magazine as one of the top ten eco-friendly restaurants in America. Seaver is an explorer for the National Geographic Society and also works as the Director of the Healthy and Sustainable Food Program at the Center for Health and the Global Environment, Harvard T.H. Chan School of Public Health. The contributing seafood editor at *Coastal Living* magazine, his work has also been featured in *Cooking Light, O: The Oprah Magazine, Every Day with Rachael Ray*, Martha Stewart's *Whole Living*, the *Washington Post*, and *Fortune*, among many others. He has also appeared on CNN, NPR, and *20/20*. Seaver was the host of the national television program *In Search of Food* on the Ovation Network and *Eat: The History of Food* on National Geographic TV.

ACKNOWLEDGMENTS

So many people have been generous with their time in the preparation of this book. I have been using seagreens for more than a decade in my kitchens, although my recent deep dive into the culture and science of this wonderful culinary opportunity has been energized by many who have been generous in sharing their knowledge, in some cases a lifetime of it. Though there are too many to name here, I would like to thank Bren Smith, Katy Rivera, Maine Fresh Sea Farms, Peter Arnold, Peter Fischer, Seth Barker, Barry Costa-Pierce, Maine Coast Sea Vegetables, Seraphina Erhart, Maine SeaGrant, Charlie Yarish, John Boos and Co., Staub, Zwilling-Henkels, and Vitamix.

INDEX

A

Algae species, 12–17
Alginates, 26
Alginic acid (alginato), 104
Amino acids, protein and, 28–29
Anchovies, about, 38, 82
Antioxidants, free radicals and, 96
Antioxidants, seagreens and, 92
Apples
  Arugula, Mint, Apple, and Seagreens Salad, 99
  Sautéed Seagreens with Bacon, Apple, and Onion, 91
  Seagreens Braised Collard Style with Apple Cider, 96
Arsenic precaution, 119
Artichokes, in Seagreen and Artichoke Dip, 70
Arugula, Mint, Apple, and Seagreens Salad, 99
Asparagus and Dulse Quiche with Goat Cheese, 66–67
Asparagus, white vs. green, 67
Avocados
  about: nutritional/health benefits, 58
  Choco-cado (smoothie), 61
  Seagreen Guacamole, 72

B

Bacon, in Sautéed Seagreens with Bacon, Apple, and Onion, 91
Bacon, in Shelling Bean Soup, 118
Barley, about, 37
Basil, about, 40
Bay leaf, about, 40–41
Beans and other legumes
  about: canned, preparing and salt content, 38–39, 116; rinsing, 116; soaking, 116
  Breakfast Burrito, 66
  Fiery-Hot Butter Bean and Escarole Soup, 120–121
  Lentil Soup, 117
  Minestrone, 117–118
  Moorish Stew, 123

Roasted Squash Hummus with Crunchy Wakame, 80–81
  Shelling Bean Soup, 118
  Veggie Burger, 132
Beef, in Lasagna, 128–129
Beef, in Umami-Spiked Burger, 133
Beer with seagreens, 133
Beets
  Beet and Seagreen Salad, 107
  Tomato-Veggie drink, 62
  Veggie Burger, 132
Berries
  Basic Seagreen Smoothie, 58
  Mixed Fruit Super Green (smoothie), 59
  Nut Butter and Jelly (smoothie), 60
Bladderwrack. See Rockweed
Blanching seagreens, 48
Blancmange, 138–139
Blenders, 33–34
Blood pressure elevation, seagreen intake and, 143
Blood-thinning medications, seagreens and, 143
Bloody Mary, 63
Bok choy
  Seagreen Vegetable Soup, 120
  Stir-Fried Seagreens, 127
Bonito flakes, 112
Braised Red Cabbage with Seagreens, 97
Breads, muffins, and desserts, 135–139. See also Flatbreads
  about: overview of, 135
  Blancmange, 138–139
  Chocolate Cake, 138
  Morning Glory Muffins, 136–137
  Seashore Panzanella, 107
  Seeded Multigrain Bread, 135–136
  Zucchini-Seagreen Bread, 137–138
Breakfast, 55–67. See also Drinks; Smoothies
  Asparagus and Dulse Quiche with Goat Cheese, 66–67
  Breakfast Burrito, 66
  Frittata with Sweet Potato and Sea Lettuce, 67

Kelp and Feta Omelet, 65
Spiced Nut and Seagreens Granola, 64–65
Breast health, seagreens and, 83
Bren's story (of GreenWave), 7–9
Broiled Cauliflower with Mint, Seagreens, and Parmesan, 92
Broths. See Soups, stews, and stocks
Bullwhip kelp, about, 14
Burgers, 132, 133
Burrito, breakfast, 66
Buttermilk, Kelp, and Mint Dressing, 83
Butternut squash. See Squash
Butter sauce, seagreen, 86
Buying seagreens
  fresh, 47
  frozen, 47–48
  general guidelines, 46–47
  sources for, 46–47, 144
  storing after, 144–145
  volume/price vs. farmed (land) greens, 48

C

Cabbage
  about: slaw without, 104
  Braised Red Cabbage with Seagreens, 97
  Stir-Fried Seagreens, 127
Cake, chocolate, 138
Calcium, 7, 22–23, 25–26, 142
Caldo (Sea) Verde, 115
Calories from seagreens, 31
Cancer, seagreens and, 143
Caponata, butternut squash and seagreen, 90–91
Caramelized Onions with Kombu (flatbread), 75
Carrageenan, 16, 26, 148
Carrots, in Fennel, Carrot, and Seagreens Salad, 102–103
Carrots, in Moroccan Salad, 104
Cauliflower, broiled with mint, seagreens, and parmesan, 92
Celery Root Slaw with Seagreens, 104

Cheese
    about: paneer, 126
    Dulse-Speckled Goat Cheese, 73
    eggs with. *See Eggs*
    Saag Paneer, 126–127
Cherries, in Mixed Fruit Super Green
    (smoothie), 59
Cherry Mint (smoothie), 60
Chervil, about, 41
Chicken
    Chicken and Seagreen Stock, 113
    Dashi-Braised Chicken with Root
        Vegetables, 125–126
    Lasagna, 128–129
    Seafood or Chicken Chile Verde, 131
Chili verde, seafood or chicken, 131
Chips, seagreen, 69, 146
Chocolate and cacao
    Choco-cado (smoothie), 61
    Chocolate Cake, 138
Cilantro, about, 41
Coconut, in Piña Colada (smoothie), 61
Cooking with seagreens
    about: overview of, 45–46
    amount to use (fresh/frozen/hydrated),
        49
    blanching, 48
    buying and. *See Buying seagreens*
    cooking times, 52
    flavor extraction, 52
    fresh vs. frozen, 47–48, 147
    general guidelines, 51
    getting family to eat seagreens and, 147
    main courses and, 51
    questions/answers on, 146–147
    rehydrating seagreens, 49–50, 147
    smoking tips/insights, 53
    storing and, 144–145
    types of seagreen to use, 51, 146
Corn and cornmeal
    about: cornmeal, 38
    Furikake Seasoned Popcorn, 70–71
    Polenta with Seagreens and Parmesan,
        94
    Summer Corn Salad, 100
Crackers, multigrain, 71–72
Creamed Seagreens, 95
Creole Grill Seasoning, 87
Cucumber, in Gazpacho, 114
Cucumber, in Spicy Smashed Cucumber
    with Candied Ginger, 102
Curry sauce, 85
Cutting board, 33

D
Dairy products, seagreens and, 70
Desserts. *See Breads, muffins, and desserts*

Detoxification, seagreens and, 143–144
Dill, about, 41–42
Dips
    Seagreen and Artichoke Dip. *See Snacks*
    Seagreen Guacamole, 72
Diseases/conditions, aided by seagreens,
    143
Drinks. *See also Smoothies*
    about: beer with seagreens, 133; black tea
        and green tea, 64; juices, fiber, and sugar
        absorption, 62; teas and tisanes, 63
    Bloody Mary, 63
    Tomato-Veggie, 62
    Wellness Tea, 64
Drying processes, for seagreens, 142
Dulse, about, 16

E
Eggs
    Asparagus and Dulse Quiche with Goat
        Cheese, 66–67
    Frittata with Sweet Potato and Sea
        Lettuce, 67
    Kelp and Feta Omelet, 65
Electrolytes, 30
Energy bars, 73
Entrées. *See Larger dishes*
Equipment, kitchen, 33–35
Escarole, in Fiery-Hot Butter Bean and
    Escarole Soup, 120–121

F
FAQs. *See Questions/answers on seagreens*
Farming seagreens, 5, 6, 7–9
Fennel
    about, 103
    Fennel, Carrot, and Seagreens Salad,
        102–103
    Seagreens with Italian Fennel Salad, 109
Fiber, 31, 62, 142

Fiery-Hot Butter Bean and Escarole Soup,
    120–121
Fish. *See Seafood*
Flatbreads, 74–75
    Caramelized Onions with Kombu, 75
    Flatbread with Butternut Squash and
        Smoked Dulse, 74–75
    Grilled Garlic Nori Bread, 75
    Oven-Baked Flatbread, 74
    Stovetop Flatbread, 74
Folate, 20, 21
Forests of seagreens, 6
Frozen seagreen cubes, 59
Fruit, frozen, 56. *See also Smoothies*
Fucus vesiculosus (rockweed), about, 3
Furikake Seasoned Popcorn, 70–71

G
Garlic
    about: complementing seagreens, 114;
        preparing, 39
    Grilled Garlic Nori Bread, 75
Gazpacho, 114
Ginger, in Kelp, Walnut, and Ginger Pesto,
    79–80
Ginger, preparing, 39
Granola, spiced nut and seagreen, 64–65
Grapes, in Seashore Panzanella, 107
Gravy, tangy spice, 84–85
Green bean soup, Southern-style, 119
GreenWave, evolution of, 8–9
Gremolata, smoky dulse, 84
Grilled Garlic Nori Bread, 75
Grilling, wrapping fish/chicken for, 132
Growing, 145–146
Growth, of seagreens, 11
Guacamole, seagreen, 72

H
Health-related questions/answers,
    143–144
Heavy metals, 26, 148
Herbes de Provence, 87
Herbs and spices, 39. *See also Seasoning salts;
    specific herbs and spices*
    about: personalities of, 40
    black pepper value, 72
    chopping fresh herbs, 43
    dried vs. fresh herbs, 41
    limes with herbs, 39
    seagreen-friendly herbs, 40–43
Hummus, roasted with crunchy wakame,
    80–81

I
Industry, seagreens, 6
Inflammation-reducing properties, 144
Ingredients. *See also Cooking with seagreens;
    specific main ingredients*
    herbs (seagreen-friendly), 40–43
    pantry items, 36–39
Iodine, 11, 16, 24, 53, 142, 144, 148
Irish moss, 15–16
Iron, 20, 25, 142

J
Japanese mandoline, 35
Juices. *See Drinks*

K
Kathy's Multigrain Crackers, 71–72
Kelp, types and characteristics, 12–14
Kitchen tools, 33–35
Knives, 35

L

Larger dishes, 125–133
  about: overview of, 125
  Dashi-Braised Chicken with Root
    Vegetables, 125–126
  Lasagna, 128–129
  Orecchiette with Sausage, Sweet Potatoes,
    and Seagreens, 130
  Saag Paneer, 126–127
  Seafood or Chicken Chile Verde, 131
  Stir-Fried Seagreens, 127
  Umami-Spiked Burger, 133
  Veggie Burger, 132
  Zucchini and Seagreens "Spaghetti" with
    Garlic, 129
Laver (nori), about, 16–17
Lentil Soup, 117

M

Magnesium, 25, 143
Main dishes. *See Larger dishes*
Mandoline, Japanese, 35
Manganese, 25–26
Mango
  Basic Seagreen Smoothie, 58
  Mango Margarita, 59
Mango Margarita, 59
Marinades. *See Sauces, spreads, and
  marinades*
Melatonin, 26
Metals, heavy, 148
Metals, heavy, preventing absorption of,
  26
Minerals, 22, 24–30. *See also specific minerals*
  recommended daily allowance (RDA),
    25
  vitamins vs., 142
  whole food vs. supplements, 29
Mint
  about: forms, uses, and virtues, 60
  Arugula, Mint, Apple, and Seagreens
    Salad, 99
  Buttermilk, Kelp, and Mint Dressing, 83
  Cherry Mint (smoothie), 60
  Seagreen and Herb Marinade, 81
  Shamrock Shake, 59
Mirin, 37
Miso, about, 122
Miso Soup, 122
Mixed Fruit Super Green (smoothie), 59
Moorish Stew, 123
Morning Glory Muffins, 136–137
Moroccan Salad, 104
MSG and umami, 14
Multigrain bread, seeded, 135–136
Mushrooms, enoki, in Miso Soup, 122
Mustard types, 38

N

Nori, about, 16–17
Nutrients, 19–31. *See also Protein; specific
  vitamins and minerals*
  about: vitamins vs. minerals, 27
  amount to eat: overview of, 19
  electrolytes, 30
  fiber, 31, 62, 142
  melatonin, 26
  minerals, 22, 24–30, 142
  omega fatty acids, 30–31, 58, 82
  polymers, 26–27
  questions/answers on, 142–143
  sterols, 30
  vitamins, 19–24, 142
Nutritional benefits, evolving story of, 17.
    See also Resources
Nuts and seeds
  about: to add to smoothies, 58; oils from,
    37; to stock, 37
  Kelp and Cashew Pesto, 80
  Kelp, Walnut, and Ginger Pesto, 79–80
  Moroccan Salad, 104
  Nut Butter and Jelly (smoothie), 60
  Protein Punch (smoothie), 61
  Seagreen Energy Bars, 73
  Seeded Multigrain Bread, 135–136
  Spiced Nut and Seagreens Granola,
    64–65
  Stir-Fried Seagreens, 127
  Veggie Burger, 132

O

Oats
  Kathy's Multigrain Crackers, 71–72
  Protein Punch (smoothie), 61
  Spiced Nut and Seagreens Granola,
    64–65
Oils, 36, 37
Olive oil, 37
Omega fatty acids, 30–31, 58, 82
Onions
  about: green (scallions), 42
  Caramelized Onions with Kombu
    (flatbread), 75
  Kelp, Turnip, and Sweet Onion Salad,
    109
  Sautéed Seagreens with Bacon, Apple,
    and Onion, 91
  Orecchiette with Sausage, Sweet Potatoes,
    and Seagreens, 130
Oregano (dried), about, 42

P

Pans, 34, 35
Pantry items, 36–39
Panzanella, seashore, 107

Parsley
  about, 42
  Seagreen and Herb Marinade, 81
(Sea)green Goddess Dressing, 82
Parsnips, in Minestrone, 117–118
Pasta
  about: whole wheat, 37
  Lasagna, 128–129
  Orecchiette with Sausage, Sweet Potatoes,
    and Seagreens, 130
  sauces for. *See Sauces, spreads, and marinades*
  Zucchini and Seagreens "Spaghetti" with
    Garlic, 129
Peach Melba, 61
Pear and Herbs over Seagreens Salad, 106
Pepper grinders, 35
Peppers, in Seafood or Chicken Chile
    Verde, 131
Pestos, 79–80
Phosphorus, 26
Pho with Shrimp, 121
Phycopolymers, 26–27
Pineapple, in Basic Seagreen Smoothie, 58
Pineapple, in Piña Colada (smoothie), 61
Polenta with Seagreens and Parmesan, 94
Polymers, 26–27
Popcorn, furikake seasoned, 70–71
Potassium, 27–28, 143
Potatoes
  Caldo (Sea) Verde, 115
  Dashi-Braised Chicken with Root
    Vegetables, 125–126
  Moorish Stew, 123
Protein, 28–29
  amino acids and, 28–29
  complete vs. incomplete, 29
  non-meat complete, 29
  quantity in seagreens, 29, 143
Protein Punch (smoothie), 61

Q

Questions/answers on seagreens, 141–149
  basic information, 141–142
  choosing/buying/storing seagreens,
    144–145
  cooking with seagreens, 146–147
  growing seagreens, 145–146
  health-related, 143–144
  nutrient-related, 142–143
  safety-related, 148–149
Quinoa
  about: history and characteristics, 105;
    nutritional benefits, 37; preparing, 37, 105
  Costal Quinoa Tabbouleh, 106
  Crunchy Quinoa, Sweet Potato, and
    Seagreens, 105
  Seagreen Energy Bars, 73

R

Radiation concerns, 149

Raisins

about: golden, 38; pre-salad treatment
for, 38

Morning Glory Muffins, 136–137

Moroccan Salad, 104

Raw diet, seagreens and, 146

Rehydrating seagreens, 49–50, 147

Resources, 46–47, 150–151

Rice

about: brown vs. white, 37

Umami-Rich Rice Pilaf, 94–95

Veggie Burger, 132

Roasted Squash Hummus with Crunchy
Wakame, 80–81

Rockweed, about, 3, 14–15

Rubs. *See Seasoning salts*

S

Saag Paneer, 126–127

Safety considerations, 49, 119, 148–149

Salads, 99–109

about: overview of, 99; two ways seagreens
used in, 99

Arugula, Mint, Apple, and Seagreens
Salad, 99

Beet and Seagreen Salad, 107

Celery Root Slaw with Seagreens, 104

Costal Quinoa Tabbouleh, 106

Crunchy Quinoa, Sweet Potato, and
Seagreens, 105

Fennel, Carrot, and Seagreens Salad,
102–103

Kelp, Turnip, and Sweet Onion Salad,
109

Moroccan Salad, 104

Pear and Herbs over Seagreens Salad,
106

Seagreens Sushi Joint–Style Salad,
108–109

Seagreens with Italian Fennel Salad, 109

Seashore Panzanella, 107

Sea Smoky Mediterranean Salad, 101

Spicy Smashed Cucumber with Candied
Ginger, 102

Summer Corn Salad, 100

Watermelon Salad with Lime, Mint, and
Nori, 100–101

Salt, types and flavors, 39, 88–89. *See also
Seasoning salts*

Sauces, spreads, and marinades

about: hot sauce, 37; mirin, 37;
mustard types, 38; overview of, 79;
Worcestershire sauce, 38

Buttermilk, Kelp, and Mint Dressing,
83

Kelp and Cashew Pesto, 80

Kelp, Walnut, and Ginger Pesto, 79–80

Roasted Squash Hummus with Crunchy
Wakame, 80–81

Seagreen and Herb Marinade, 81

Seagreen Butter Sauce, 86

(Sea)green Curry Sauce, 85

(Sea)green Goddess Dressing, 82

Smoky Dulse Gremolata, 84

Tangy Spice Gravy, 84–85

Toasted Nori Vinaigrette, 83

Umami-Spicy Marinara Sauce, 86

Sausage, orecchiette with sweet potatoes,
seagreens and, 130

Sautéed Seagreens with Bacon, Apple, and
Onion, 91

Seafood

about: anchovies (canned), 38, 82; sardines
(canned), 38

Caldo (Sea) Verde, 115

Pho with Shrimp, 121

Seafood or Chicken Chile Verde, 131

Spicy Fish Rub, 87

Seagreens

about: overview of varieties, 11, 141

amount to eat/adding to diet, 11, 52, 146

antioxidants and, 92

author's perspective, vi–vii

Bren's story (of GreenWave), 7–9

calories from, 31

carbon dioxide use and, 5–6

coastal cookouts and, 3

common species, 12–17. *See also specific
varieties*

cooking with. See Cooking with seagreens

dairy products and, 70

drying processes, 142

edibility of, 141

FAQs. See Questions/answers on
seagreens

farmed (land) greens vs., 48

farming, 5, 6, 7–9

forests of, 6

global industry for, 6

growing, 145–146

growth of, 11

health-related questions, 143–144

introducing into diet, 52

many uses of, 2–3, 4

nutritional/health benefits, 3–4, 7–8,
127, 141

prevalence of, 2–4

rehydrating, 49–50, 147

resources, 46–47, 150–151

safety of, 49, 148–149

"seaweed" taboo and, 1–2

storing, 144–145

sustainability and production, 4–6

taste of, 141

terminology for, 141

type to use in dishes, 51

Seagreen-wrapped root vegetables, 130

Sea lettuce, about, 17

Seashore Panzanella, 107

Sea Smoky Mediterranean Salad, 101

Seasoning salts

about: overview of, 87; types of salts for,
88–89

Creole Grill Seasoning, 87

Herbes de Provence, 87

Sicilian Herb Rub, 87

Spicy Fish Rub, 87

Seeds. *See Nuts and seeds*

Selenium, 29

Sesame oil, 37

Shamrock Shake, 59

Shelling Bean Soup, 118

Sicilian Herb Rub, 87

Side dishes, 90–97

Braised Red Cabbage with Seagreens,
97

Broiled Cauliflower with Mint,
Seagreens, and Parmesan, 92

Butternut Squash and Seagreen Caponata,
90–91

Creamed Seagreens, 95

Crispy Zucchini Cakes with Kelp and
Cashew Pesto, 93

Polenta with Seagreens and Parmesan,
94

Sautéed Seagreens with Bacon, Apple,
and Onion, 91

Seagreens Braised Collard Style with
Apple Cider, 96

Umami-Rich Rice Pilaf, 94–95

Smoke, seagreens and, 53

Smoky Dulse Chips, 69

Smoky Dulse Gremolata, 84

Smoothies

about: amount of seagreens to use, 49;
blender for, 33–34; extras for, 58;
frozen fruit for, 56; frozen seagreen
cubes for, 59; making, 57; planning
ahead for, 55–57; seagreens to use, 55,
57; soaking seagreens for, 57

Basic Seagreen Smoothie, 58

Cherry Mint, 60

Choco-cado, 61

Mango Margarita, 59

Mixed Fruit Super Green, 59

Nut Butter and Jelly, 60

Peach Melba, 61

Piña Colada, 61

Protein Punch, 61

Shamrock Shake, 59
Snacks, 69–75. See also Flatbreads
  about: making chips crisp, 146; overview of, 69; sushi, 76
  Dulse-Speckled Goat Cheese, 73
  Furikake Seasoned Popcorn, 70–71
  Kathy's Multigrain Crackers, 71–72
  Seagreen and Artichoke Dip, 70
  Seagreen Energy Bars, 73
  Seagreen Guacamole, 72
  Smoky Dulse Chips, 69
Sodium, 30, 62, 118, 122, 143
Soups, stews, and stocks, 111–123
  about: amount of seagreens to use, 49; bonito flakes with, 112; broths, 111; overview of, 111; rehydrating seagreens for, 50, 147
  Aromatic Dashi Broth, 112
  Basic Dashi Broth, 111
  Caldo (Sea) Verde, 115
  Chicken and Seagreen Stock, 113
  Fiery-Hot Butter Bean and Escarole Soup, 120–121
  Gazpacho, 114
  Lentil Soup, 117
  Minestrone, 117–118
  Miso Soup, 122
  Moorish Stew, 123
  Pho with Shrimp, 121
  Seagreen Vegetable Soup, 120
  Shelling Bean Soup, 118
  Southern-Style Green Bean Soup, 119
  Vegetable and Seagreen Broth, 113
Southern-Style Green Bean Soup, 119
Spatulas, 34
Spheres, making, 104
Spicy Fish Rub, 87
Spicy Smashed Cucumber with Candied Ginger, 102
Spinach, in Mango Margarita, 59
Spinach, in Saag Paneer, 126–127
Spirulina, about, 13
Squash
  Butternut Squash and Seagreen Caponata, 90–91
  Crispy Zucchini Cakes with Kelp and

Cashew Pesto, 93
  Flatbread with Butternut Squash and Smoked Dulse, 74–75
  Roasted Squash Hummus with Crunchy Wakame, 80–81
  Zucchini and Seagreens "Spaghetti" with Garlic, 129
  Zucchini-Seagreen Bread, 137–138
Sterols, 30
Stir-Fried Seagreens, 127
Storing seagreens, 144–145
Sugar absorption, fiber and, 63
Sugar kelp, about, 13
Summer Corn Salad, 100
Sushi, seagreens and, 76
Sustainability of seagreens, 5
Sweet potatoes
  Crunchy Quinoa, Sweet Potato, and Seagreens, 105
  Frittata with Sweet Potato and Sea Lettuce, 67
  Orecchiette with Sausage, Sweet Potatoes, and Seagreens, 130

T
Tabbouleh, coastal quinoa, 106
Tarragon, about, 43
Tarragon, in (Sea)green Goddess Dressing, 82
Teas and tisanes. See Drinks
Thyme, about, 43
Toasted Nori Vinaigrette, 83
Tomatoes
  about: canned fire-roasted, 38
  Bloody Mary, 63
  Gazpacho, 114
  Tomato-Veggie drink, 62
  Umami-Spicy Marinara Sauce, 86
Tools, kitchen, 33–35
Turkey, in Lasagna, 128–129
Turnips, 109, 125–126

U
Umami, defined, 147
Umami, MSG and, 14
Umami-Rich Rice Pilaf, 94–95

Umami-Spicy Marinara Sauce, 86
Umami-Spiked Burger, 133

V
Varieties of seagreens, 12–17. See also specific varieties
Vegetables
  about: seagreen-wrapped root veggies, 130
  Butternut Squash and Seagreen Caponata, 90–91
  Dashi-Braised Chicken with Root Vegetables, 125–126
  soups, broths with. See Soups, stews, and stocks
  Tomato-Veggie drink, 62
Veggie Burger, 132
Vinegars, 36
Vitamins
  about: fat-soluble vs. water-soluble, 23; minerals vs., 142; recommended daily allowance (RDA), 25; whole food vs. supplements, 29
  vitamin A, 12, 19
  vitamin B (B vitamins), 12, 20–21, 26, 142
  vitamin C, 7, 20, 25
  vitamin D, 12, 22, 26
  vitamin E, 23
  vitamin K, 24

W
Wakame, about, 13
Watermelon Salad with Lime, Mint, and Nori, 100–101
Weight loss, seagreens and, 142
Wellness Tea, 64
White powder, on seagreens, 144
Wine with seagreens, 128
Winged kelp, about, 12
Worcestershire sauce, 38
Workouts, nutrients after, 28
Wrapping foods with seagreens, 130, 132

Z
Zucchini. See Squash

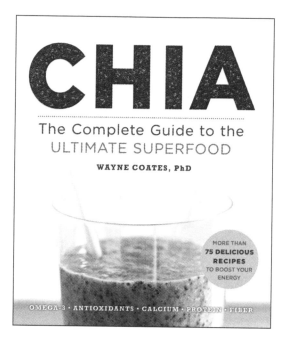

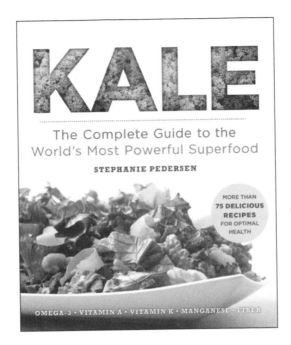

KALE

The Complete Guide to the World's Most Powerful Superfood
Stephanie Pedersen
978-1-4549-0625-4

From farmers and foodies to celebrity chefs—everyone's gone mad for kale! For those eager to get in on this healthy, tasty trend, here is a fun-to-read, one-stop resource for all things kale, including more than 75 delicious recipes to entice, satisfy, and boost well-being. Stephanie Pedersen, a holistic health counselor, provides dozens of tips for making kale delicious and desirable to even the most finicky eater.

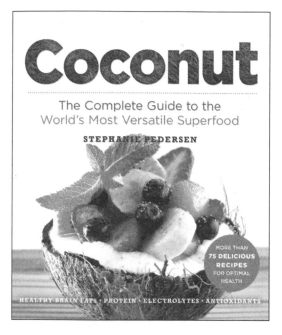

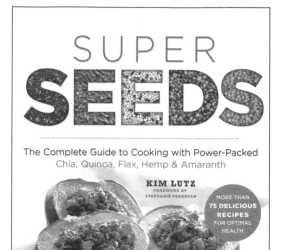

COCONUT

The Complete Guide to the
World's Most Versatile Superfood

Stephanie Pedersen

978-1-4549-1340-5

Perfect for dishes both savory and sweet, coconut is delicious—and, even better, it's a nutritional powerhouse with myriad health benefits. Find out how to choose, use, and store every bit of the coconut, along with more than 75 recipes that make you feel as good as they taste. And, in addition to informative sidebars, there's advice on making coconut-based beauty supplies!

SUPER SEEDS

The Complete Guide to Cooking with Power-Packed Chia, Quinoa, Flax, Hemp & Amaranth

Kim Lutz

978-1-4549-1278-1

Five super seeds—in one super volume! Chia, hemp, flax, quinoa, and amaranth are tiny powerhouses that deliver whopping amounts of protein, essential fatty acids, and great taste in every serving. Perfect for vegan and gluten-free diets, they're the stars of these 75 mouthwatering recipes. Essential for anyone interested in eating healthily . . . and deliciously.